Killer Breasts

A Compassionate Step-by-Step Guide to Overcome Breast Implant Illness, Cleanse Your Body, Heal Your Hormones and Ignite Your Life!

D1521110

Diane Kazer, FDN-P, HHC

Table of Contents

Foreward

I LOVE this book. This book is an accelerator. More on what I mean below.

When you notice something in your body is not functioning right and is of concern to you, what's your usual pattern?

•Avoidance? "it's not too bad, maybe it will go away by tomorrow". That may be a healthy response and keeps us from becoming a hypochondriac.

•Rationalization? "Everybody has got some kind of health issue".

•Fate? "Yes, this condition runs in the family-it's my genes"

•Grit, Determination and Will-power? "This is NOT going to take me down".

•Hopelessness? "There's nothing I can do." Or, "I've tried everything".

•Exasperation? "Ain't nobody got time for this"!

•Pharmaceutical? "If I take a couple of Advil, I have no problems with exercising".

Perhaps we know 'something's not right', but there's no clear path as to what to do. So, we ignore, or better word, compartmentalize our concern for a future day.

We all develop our own way of dealing with our bodies. After all. We have to get up and do our day. Whether it's feeding the kids, a spouse, getting to work on time, … most of us don't have the luxury to just stop our lives and give full attention to a body that isn't quite firing on all 8 cylinders (can you tell I'm a Detroit guy at heart)?

We may know deep in our hearts that 'something has got to change', but 'it's not that bad', or you have no idea what to do, and our immediate life-demands take up our time and awareness.

Most Health Care Practitioners have wrestled with the question again and again "why doesn't this patient get it? Why don't they understand the danger of the situation? How can I say it differently for them to understand, accept and then take action"? The answer for me to this conundrum came in the 1994 'game-changer' classic by James Prochaska and team 'Changing For Good'. In the book, they broke it down into identifying the different stages we go through when some information rocks our boat too much.

•Pre-contemplation is the stage at which there is no intention to change behavior in the foreseeable future. Many individuals in this stage are unaware or under-aware of their problems." Some people call this phase "denial."

I call it the "I'm fine" syndrome. We live in a world today full of deflection, avoidance, and lack of connection with others. Our Sociologists tells us as a society we are more disconnected from community living, more isolated in our own private worlds than ever before in history. Over the years I've noticed when I ask someone "How are you", and they respond "I'm fine, how are you", I often have no clue how that person is doing, it's a convenient deflection. Therapists tell us the word F.I.N.E often means Frightened, Insecure, Neurotic and Emotional. Imagine you're seeing a neighbor at the grocery store who you haven't seen in a few weeks. When you say "Hey Steve, how are you", which is more satisfying to you as an answer? "I'm fine, how are you", or "It's a good day today, how's your day going"? I submit the second type of response gives a positive spin on the interaction, and gives a spoonful of good-will to your fellow man. Pre-contemplation is the stage of having blinders on, being unable to fully see what's in front of you. And we all have this to some degree

•Contemplation is the stage in which people are aware that a problem exists and are seriously thinking about overcoming it but have not yet made a commitment to take action. Many people in this stage can be described as ambivalent. They want to improve their blood sugar, but are not yet ready to cut back on eating sweets.

•The Preparation stage can be considered the information gathering and planning stage. The preparation stage is the most important. Turns out it is critically important. Fifty percent of the people who attempt behavior change and skip this stage will relapse within 21 days. 3 weeks! That's the 'New Years' Resolutions that start out with the best of intent and fizzle out. If you want to drive from Chicago to Miami, you need a map all the way there. If you think you 'know' how to get to Miami, because you've driven through Ohio, you're going to have a problem. You're good with the

3

map to Ohio, perhaps it's in your memory banks. But from there, without a map, you're likely to make wrong turns along the way. You need a map all the way to Miami. The Preparation stage (designing your map to address your health concern), is getting your ducks in a row with realistic expectations of the bumps along the way as you're changing the direction your health is going in.

•Action is the stage in which individuals modify their behaviour, experiences, or environment in order to overcome their problems. Action involves the most overt behavioral changes and requires considerable commitment of time and energy. During the action stage, one implements the plans developed and information gathered in the preparation stage. Jumping into the Action stage without preparation is like heading off on a road trip to Miami with maps that'll take you to Ohio.

•Maintenance is the stage in which people work to prevent relapse and consolidate the gains attained during action. For addictive behaviours, this stage extends from six months to an indeterminate period past the initial action."

Why am I talking about 'Change For Good' principles, and how does this relate to 'Killer Breasts'? Because in our world today, so many little girls are imprinted to grow up being some version of the Barbie doll she had as a child. Or it's opposite. Every young woman is told again and again in Social, television, magazines, and on-line media that outer beauty is the ticket to happiness. Cosmetics, flowing hair, enhancements... We all know this story. It's the norm in the U.S.

Yet a global report about beauty (in women) surveyed men and women in 27 countries, from Saudi Arabia and Canada to Brazil and South Africa. The results can be summarised by a quote from Audrey Hepburn: "True beauty in a woman is reflected in her soul."

According to this survey, the citizens of the world think happiness, kindness, confidence, humor and intelligence are more important than the appearance of your skin, the shape of your body or face, your hairstyle or your make-up . Quite different than the messaging a child receives in the U.S.

'Killer Breasts' is the first-hand experience from a woman who first denied, then became aware, then suffered and cried, walked, cried, crawled, screamed in anger, got up again and started walking some more, through all 5 Stages of 'Change For Good' on the topic of implantations (breasts, buttocks, Botox...). I've known Diane for a number of years and been a behind-the-scenes friend empowering her often-emotionally painful and unfortunately all-too-common journey from Double D's and temporary nirvana (pre-contemplation) through dis-ease (contemplation), to Functional Medicine deep dives (Preparation), through the ups and downs of Action, into Maintenance and carrying this message out to the world. I can think of no better Coach, and no better Advocate, for those learning about the life-threatening dangers of implants than Diane Kazer and her book 'Killer Breasts'. Reading this book gives you the map to get all the way to your Miami of abundant, vibrant health. Get ready, a paradigm shift is on your horizon.

Dr. Tom O'Bryan

www.theDr.com

Dedication

I dedicate this book to you, my sister in BII suffering. I see your pain, beauty and COURAGE to walk through it all.

I also dedicate this book to one of my greatest teachers, my mother.

In this life, I have hated you, cherished you, traveled with you, adored you, wanted to be you, cried with you, threw massive fits at you, shamed you, judged you, accused you, hid from you, lied to you, blamed you, yelled at you, felt victimized by you, tried to gain approval from you...and through it all...you still loved me, and have always stood by my side.

You emptied my blood drains after my surgery and cared for me when I was weak.

What I didn't realize as a child, but what I do now...is how I was treating you had nothing to do with you...it had EVERYTHING to do with how I was treating me. Shame projected outward as blame. What a powerful journey this has been to GET to learn this through you.

Our relationship has inspired much of the work I refer to in this book and beyond in addressing 'The Mother Wound' and 'The Father Wound'. "Every time I judge someone else, I reveal an unhealed part of me"...all judgment is self-judgment.

Whatever I see and dislike about you reveal the wounds I have yet to heal within myself ... and the lessons I came here to learn.

What I love about you are the things within me, I learned from you! You are a powerful mirror to reflect back to me where I still have yet to grow.

I honor your teaching me how to live... and suffering so I could witness the consequences of how NOT to live too. The sacrifice you made is unmatched with words.

Thanks for being on loan to me for a while!

I love you mama.

Intro

My neighbor, Megan knocked on my door and shouted through the front window from the porch "Diane, you wanna come over and play Barbies"?

A part of me cringed.

Another part of me wanted to play.

So, I ran out to join her.

When I got to her room, I noticed...

Megan had a new Ken doll, some kind of new edition sporty Barbie and a perky blonde Skipper.

And the whole family had a new red Corvette.

Perhaps not so ironically, Megan's mom just got one too and it was in the driveway.

I'll never forget that day.

The level of anger and rage I felt moved me to resent the dolls that lay before me.

Perfectly shaped in their anorexic form.

I observed the perma' smiles on their face, with bleach white teeth, bleach white, shiny hair and bright pink lipstick

What the actual fuck?

It was my first potent experience with deep shame of anticipated failure as a teenage Barbie.

How could I ever compete with Skipper?

9

She's always smiling.

Tits perked up into her chin.

Sparkly everything and a Ken doll who never leaves her.

This isn't real.

This was the first time I felt my warrior within, step up to protect me from an illusion.

That part of me that felt compelled to destroy the impossible set of standards before me.

The next thing I knew, I looked around to witness the war zone I created.

Plastic legs and arms strewn across the floor.

I gazed down at Barbie's face as I smashed it together, with my fingers.

"There, now you're not so perfect looking".

Megan looked up at me and asked, in a disturbed voice "What are you doing"?

I can only answer now what I know my then self was thinking.

I'm pulling apart a cultural narrative that shapes the illusion of happiness through a falsely idealized perfect body, face, car, daughter, husband masked with "toxic beauty".

It was though a part of me knew the weed was planted that in order to be happy I had to be beautiful and that part of me was also resentful at that unrealistic formula I would never be able to attain. The not enough'itis belief was planted and pop culture fertilized it with every exposure to perfect women who got all the fame and attention - Pamela Anderson, Playboy, Baywatch – the programming persisted, and it was everywhere I looked.

I never put her parts back together.

But metaphorically, Barbie that day.... represented the me that was to come.

This is the Humpty Dumpty story I love so much that represents us all. This BII experience is our great fall. As the story goes, we got breast implants, they were too top heavy for us to balance on the wall for too long, so we fell off and broke into a million tiny pieces. We stood up, looked around at the mess, labeled ourselves as 'broken', then went from doctor to expert, friend to guru asking them to please put us back together again. Yet, the blessing and the curse is this: Only YOU can put yourself back together again. And this book is your guide to help you do that, by understanding the pieces that make up you as a whole, which is why I go so deep into helping you really grasp the magnificence that you are.

The Japanese have a theory that goes like this: You are more beautiful for having been broken! Kintsugi is built on the concept of finding the strength and beauty in imperfection. When a ceramic object breaks, the kintsugi technique uses gold dust and to reattach the broken pieces. The resulting piece is assembled intentionally incorporating the unique cracks into its design, and the gold lines add to the beauty of the piece while strengthening it.

11

By repairing broken ceramics it's possible to give a new lease of life to pottery that becomes even more refined thanks to its "scars". The Japanese art of kintsugi teaches that broken objects are not something to hide but to display with pride. And this is the intention I have for you in this book, my friend!

My intention for you and How to Use this Book:

By the end of this book, I want you to feel confident in your understanding of these questions:

- Who do I talk to?
- What doctor can I trust?
- How do I know it's my implants causing me symptoms?
- What if I remove my implants and don't get better? Will I regret it?
- What are my options with explant and breast revisions?
- Can I still remove my 'killer breasts' and have beautiful natural ones?
- How much will it cost?
- How do I talk to my loved ones about this?
- What are all the steps I absolutely must take prior to explant?
- How do I heal and detox my body post explant?
- Who am I without my implants? I'm scared others won't think I'm beautiful and they'll ... leave me? Judge me? Feel sorry for me. Bully me!
- Will I feel beautiful without them?
- How do I do all of this without losing my mind?

- Or is this all in my head?

- I wish there was ONE resource that could help me with all of this, is there one?

YES! Yes, there is. And you've found it!

When I intuitively knew it was largely my implants making me sick, I made a promise to my body. My mind negotiated a deal with my then toxic temple... "If we take this journey and take one for the team to understand everything possible about how breast implants impact our body from all angles, then learn how to heal from breast implant illness, we will write a book to share the formula with women who are where we are right now, deal?"

To which my body replied "DEAL! But let's make this fast, we can't handle too much more of this pain. I'll give you everything I've got to give you time to research everything you can".

Then my soul chimed in "We've got this. This is the heart work we came here to share with the world! From silicone to sovereignty, suffering to self-love, do not remove your implants until you've learned the lesson you got them to teach you. Then designed the formula to help others free themselves".

On my knees, I cried and thanked spirit for the opportunity to experience this pain so that it would become my purpose!

I wrote this book to help women who truly wish to uncover the truth, recover their natural beauty, and discover their souls calling!

This book is a combination of a gift from my soul and the science that has finally been revealed to us regarding the truth about breast implants. My soul goal is to help every woman understand the toxic implications of having breast implants, the possible conditions, symptoms and suffering that may arise from having them...and how to identify the difference of, whether it's your implants making you sick or if it's something else.

Whether or not a woman decides to remove her ex plant her breast implants, is a very personal decision. And it may take her some time to come to terms with the fact that her breast implants are a key root cause, making her sick and causing side effects.

My intention is to assist her along the journey from asking the question, if her breast implants are making her sick to making the decision to explant and beyond. She will have a roadmap, on what to do to cleanse her body heal her hormones address gut infections and ignite her life.

The tools that we'll use along the journey will be advanced diagnostic labs, so she'll know exactly what to ask her doctor, or her alternative health care practitioner. To assess where she's at with her hormones, her gut health toxicity levels, and potential sources for environmental toxins. In addition to breast implants. She will also realize all of the areas, causing her toxicity, not limited to breast implants.

I wanted to thank all of the BII groups, doctors, researchers, organizations, support groups and explant warriors for being a beacon of light for the millions of women, including myself, that are searching for answers where the medical community had none.

There is a lot of conflicting data on everything from labs and supplements to surgery approaches to surgeons, so my goal is to simplify that for you as much as possible.

I also hold space for a day where every soul who stands up to offer a new way, method, solution is honored, and extended heart felt gratitude to, for their service to women suffering from BII, rather than shamed and criticized, accused of 'taking advantage of sick women'. Women who have grown sick from this, are by definition, victims of toxicity and trauma, so it is vital we use this experience to end our victim narrative, by seeing the silver lining in our suffering, as a wakeup call to wise up!

I can only speak for myself that I have invested over 10 hours per day nearly every day for 2+ years learning everything I could about BII, and prior to that learning the foundations of health, fitness, yoga, nutrition, mental wellness, functional medicine, holistic health, environmental toxicity, and more.

I am in awe for all of the wellness warriors who have paved the way for all of us to learn about something that I believe will save the lives of every woman who has breast implants in her beautiful body, blocking her sacred heart.

My recommendation is to have a journal handy, as you read this book, to document your symptoms, challenges, goals, dreams so that you can formulate an action plan. I also have a Resources section on my website for shortcuts, links and solutions that are updated regularly. I did not include them in this book since they are constantly evolving, and I wanted you to have easy access to a source where everything is updated as the science unfolds. You will also find checklists to print out for what to ask your doctor, toxic survey scores, and more!

You can find it here: www.dianekazer.com/resources

My wish for you after reading this book is to feel at peace, understood and empowered. While it is impossible to customize this journey to every women in one book, I trust you will discover the answers you have been searching for without having to scour the internet, see more doctors, or run more labs than you have to.

Also, if you make the call to keep your breast implants, yay for that too. I just want you to feel 100% confident and certain in whatever you decide. Although breast implants impact every woman differently, I will always hold the belief they are not safe in any woman's body, but that is your own personal choice. If you keep them, I do recommend you double down on your cleansing strategies, routines, supplements, hacks as well as hormone, gut, brain and lymphatic drainage support. I still support women who have breast implants, run their labs, create customized protocols...but sometimes part of my protocol is to explant, because I can see how they are impacting her body through my analysis.

You are not crazy. You're not alone. And you are about to endure one of the most awakening experiences of your life. I do believe this journey will provide you the confidence you were originally after when you got breast implants.

You ready?

Let's FLY!

Why do we REALLY Get Breast Implants?

"I didn't get implants because I was ashamed of my body, I got them to feel more confident about myself".

What has driven us all to get implants is not to 'get more confidence'.

Sure, we all want to boost self-esteem.

And the easy track to that is to do what 'they' say 'should' make us feel more beautiful, confident, sexy, worthy.

The cultural messages flashed before our eyes are a form of gaslighting that lights the fire of shame within our ego.

One billboard says 'Love your body as it is' and embedded in the same message is 'But you need to buy our product to feel better about yourself' with an image of a celebrity that got photoshopped for 2 hours.

It's not our fault.

You weren't born this way.

You were culturally conditioned this way.

The root of our desire to amend our bodies and cut ourselves open obsessed with the unrealistic endeavor to be perfect, is shame.

Toxic Shame.

As you read this, please keep in mind that this isn't just about removing your breast implants and recovering your body to how it once was in the aftermath.

Why would you want to go backwards to the insecure woman who was not happy with herself as she was?

This book is your ticket to freedom. Transformation. Warrior fuel.

A new level of self-love and self-respect that no longer puts up with the prison bars of society that says a woman 'should' look this way or that.

This book is intended to challenge how you think so you stop blindly trusting organizations that care more about their wealth than your health.

I wish for this to open your mind, heart and third eye to see truth about the 'beauty industry' and ultimately the 'natural beauty' that is and has always been within YOU.

As you read each chapter, I want you to imagine with every belief, thought, story, toxin, trauma a part of your non-self falls away, getting closer and closer to the you, that is your true beauty, your real power and your inner purpose. Ask yourself 'Where else have I given my power away, by conforming to others 'shoulds'? Where else have I overinvested trust or pedestalized people – physicians, politicians, parents, peers – that they knew better than I, about my body?

Remember when healing yourself, you become a healer of others and a healer of the Planet. This is the most sacred work you will ever do!

May I also ask, that you gift a copy of this book to every woman who either desires breast implants or has them? Please also share this book with doctors, surgeons and health experts who work with patients who have them, so they know what to look out for. It's up to them what to do with it, but doesn't every woman deserve to know the truth about what could be causing her harm that she was never warned about before she installed them?

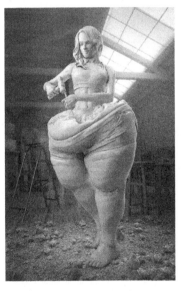

Dear beautiful sister, you are both the Sculptor and the work of art!

Chapter 1: You've Tried Everything, Your Labs Are Normal, No One Knows What's Wrong and You Feel Like You're Going Crazy!

Emily is a happily married, 35-year-old, new mom and is highly intelligent. She is powerful, with unique gifts, and she's usually unstoppable. But over the last 8 months, since she had her baby boy, she's felt like she's been failing as a mother, because she's had so little energy with such severe brain fog that it's been difficult to get much done, let alone care for her son or keep up with even minor household duties.

Emily has intuitively known for some time now that something is majorly wrong. But she can't seem to figure it out on her own. She has tried. Many symptoms. Many years. Many doctors. Many failed attempts. Living a life in pain is a life in vain with nothing to gain-- except medical bills and regret ...

She suffered from debilitating migraines, depression, anxiety, insomnia, chronic fatigue, diarrhea, constipation, muscle weakness and unexplained weight loss. She had such terrible food sensitivities, that she was down to only being able to stomach four to five foods every day. Everything else made her sick, and her body reacted with unpleasantly inflammatory symptoms such as rosacea, excessive itching, rashes and total body pain. Especially being a new mother, she was concerned for her life with heart palpitations that seemed to come out of nowhere and woke up most mornings in a puddle of sweat. "Ugh did I soak my sheets again…. I have to figure out what's really going on, I can't live like this anymore".

Since all of her blood tests came back 'perfectly normal' and she was told she was the picture of health, she did some research online and scheduled an appointment with a local naturopath.

She had allergy and food sensitivity testing done and adjusted her diet accordingly, except the small indulgences here and there. She ate consciously and stuck with low inflammatory foods. Her doctor prescribed the low histamine diet, Auto Immune Paleo and Keto diet. She felt better, but still felt 'off'. She went vegan, ate mostly organic, gluten free, dairy free…because, she wanted to be free.

Eating out became a challenge, so she just stopped going to restaurants, because why bother? She felt isolated from her friends and she mourned her social life.

She had been on juice cleanses, tried celery juice, intermittent fasting, three-day fasts… One popular detox method after another; you name it, she tried it.

Since she still felt off, she consulted with a functional medicine expert who specialized in bio-identical hormones and thyroid treatment, which made her feel somewhat normal for a couple of months, until it stopped… Nothing seemed to work-- her hormones were just completely off.

She couldn't sleep, and she felt stressed all the time. The constant struggle to get her health in order took a toll on her spirit. So, she consulted a therapist who prescribed anti-depressants. Then sleep medications. And when that didn't work, she was prescribed Xyrem to sedate her… 'date rape' drug to the rescue. She didn't want to be on all of these medications and over the counter drugs, but she felt she had no choice.

She used to be full of energy, life and motivation to get $hit done, conquer the world, exercise and socialize. But she didn't feel like doing any of that. She just wanted to crawl under the covers and scream and cry. "What TF is happening to me? Am I just supposed to accept this as my new norm? Am I just getting old? Is this what life looks like after becoming a mom?"

She was miserable, wanted to be free from her symptoms and to just feel normal again.

When I met Emily, her everyday life was consumed by frustration over her umpteen symptoms and the inability to get to the root cause. She went from doctor to doctor and ran several functional lab tests and spent tens of thousands of dollars on the best supplements, therapies and treatments but no one seemed to understand what she was going through, nor could anyone address the root cause of her problems. She was highly motivated to do whatever it took to get better, yet was having a hard time trusting me, because everything else had failed her.

And even with all of the medications she was taking to numb out her pain and anxiety, she was still experiencing a myriad of emotions such as:

Worthlessness and guilt for the burden it put on her mom and husband since she couldn't do much for her son, husband nor the house.

Helplessness and overwhelm as it felt like there were too many steps to take to get healthy and not enough time to do it.

She was afraid that nothing would work because she tried what felt like everything to get better, but nothing did…. until one day…she discovered someone that had asked her something that no one else had.

What was it that her doctors weren't asking her?

"Got breast implants?"

It's a personal question, but it's become our moral duty to ask. Millions have them, yet few are told the truth about the damage they cause.

The common woman today is laser-focused on looking and feeling younger. Yet as she carries these ticking time bombs inside her, those efforts are grossly negated. The modern-day woman is *dying* to be beautiful. With today's technology, there are much safer alternatives to breast implant reconstruction and I want to share them with you, so you can age gracefully, with self-love from the inside out and cellular health from the outside in!

I've worked with clients who developed Lupus from their implants rupturing. Multiple other clients expressed such extreme exhaustion, they couldn't get out of bed; not to mention, three of my close friends' mothers likely died from theirs.

Various findings, as well as my personal experience, show that, *every* woman who explants needs to focus on detox for at least a year. It's unknown whether silicone is even something we *can* detox completely. As many of you already know: Yes, all implants bleed, leak and / or rupture.

Women suffering from BII have different stories, but their I symptoms are evident. Would you still want breast implants if ten women sent you this list of complications they've had since they installed theirs?

"I am experiencing flu-like symptoms, numbness in my hands, arms and feet. Major sleep issues, Severe IBS – constipation! Short-term memory. Back pain, shoulder pain, fatigue, swollen eyes and thyroid problems."

"Chronic fatigue, fibromyalgia, EBV, Hashimoto's, hepatitis. Symptoms started at age twenty-seven, (so thirty-four years ago), and have gotten worse over the years."

"I have had [implants] for three years. I have had chronic hives since three weeks [post op]. I have sweating issues. I am tired all of the time. My eyes are black. I have symptoms of every autoimmune [disease]. I'm afraid they're going to kill me."

"I am bedridden after a rupture and silicone revision last year. I had symptoms for eight of my ten lovely years with these toxic pieces of life-sucking sh*t."

"I've had psoriatic arthritis for years. After implants I'm exhausted. Feels like I am slowly dying."

"My ten-month-old baby boy is sick and will no longer breast feed. It's as though he knows my milk is filled with toxic beauty chemicals, and I am left with this sense of guilt that my desire to be artificially beautiful is what poisoned him."

"My son has autism, and I can't help but to wonder if my breast implants caused or contributed to that. I'll never know but knowing what I know now about how toxic they are, I would have never gotten them, much less birthed a child with them in".

Sounds familiar, eh? But at least you have Killer Breasts. What part of us felt this was all worth it when we got them put in? Are fake boobs *that* important to sacrifice all of this?

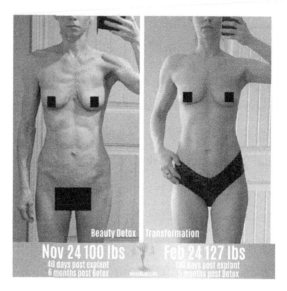

Beauty Detox | Transformation
Nov 24 100 lbs   Feb 24 127 lbs
40 days post explant   130 days post explant
6 months post Botox   5 months post Botox

After Emily had her implants removed, her health deteriorated. She had extreme estrogen dominance, high estrogen and low progesterone. Her neurotoxic levels were extremely high (take the quiz on my website). She was skin and bones, emaciated to the point of being concerned for her life. She wanted to end it. Her son was now sick, refused to breast feed and was suffering symptoms similar to her: gastrointestinal issues, skin rashes, food sensitivities, mood swings, he couldn't keep food down and she feared for his life too. My team had to step in to help them both, and while it wasn't pretty, it was necessary. Little Lyle's functional labs revealed the same infections and inflammation as his mama. Had Emily not sought support before, after and throughout, the unfortunate reality is, she may not have made it, as this constellation of symptoms from BII and Toxic Beauty are a mystery to solve even for the most well intended, famous doctors.

28

Emily had also been doing Botox injections for her migraines at the same time, so it's hard to say which of the toxins pushed her over the edge. From my own experience and research, Botox is also extremely neurotoxic to the body, being the #1 most toxic substance known to man, but that is for my next book about 'Toxic Beauty'.

For the last decade, I've been seeking health and restoration for my own body. I've gone deeper into custom nutrition, functional medicine lab testing, the importance of daily detox, advanced level bio hacks, partnering with the best of the best doctors, mindset coaches and holistic health practitioners... I'm the emblazoned picture of health on the outside, yet riddled with dis-ease on the inside. I'm that girl who won bikini competitions, but somehow lost her vitality. I started leading 'self-love' and sexy food cleanse groups years ago, before I loved myself, because I was dying inside to be loved and be beautiful.

I'm the warrior who stands up to spread truth about the toxins that lurk in our environment. Yet, until recently, *never* considered the *greatest* toxin of all, one I am exposed to every single day. The ticking time bombs that sit right over my heart, the very seat of connection, immunity and production of the most potent hormone of all, Oxytocin. Otherwise known as the 'love hormone', when it's low, Cortisol, the fear and stress hormone, is high, making it hard to breath.

It was enough to have this song stuck in my head all day, "Every breath I take, every move I make, every single day, every game I play… I'm leaking silicone!"

Now that might sound a little extreme for you… Or maybe it just sounds like a familiar song from the nineties that Biggie Smalls later remixed. Either way, it's a true story-- but not one that we've read, which makes it hard to believe. I get it. I didn't want to believe it, either.

All implants leak, bleed or rupture … Eventually. For women with implants, (and anyone with *any* silicone and/or saline implant in their body), the toxins bleed into our bodies from *day one* of implantation. Silicone, saline as well as thirty plus other toxins and heavy metals migrate to our lymph nodes, liver and brain. It doesn't happen to one, it happens to all.

This book is for all of you who have been experiencing "mysterious" symptoms that doctors can't trace the root of, which is exactly what happened to me and every other woman who experiences the side effects of implants. Clearly these warning signs can proliferate all over the body, they're not just isolated to the area of the breasts.

What may be baffling is how symptoms can seem totally unrelated. However, I can assure you, they are not! I am proof. As are countless other heroic women who listened to the call within themselves. The voice that cried, "Help." One which they were compelled to answer, in order to survive.

How did I know it was my implants? The answer is, I didn't. I realize many of my symptoms may be implant-related, and yet others can be from other things.

I started this journey to figure out what the frack was going on with my health... It was a complete mystery to me why no matter what advanced techniques, treatments or tinctures I tried on my body, nothing worked to slow the symptoms. At one point, I threw my hands up and said, "I literally have done *everything* I can for my physical, nutritional, and emotional body... There is *something wrong* inside." And deep down, my intuition whispered, "These are poisoning you. It's time to put them to rest."

Then in the midst of many bodily fluids, I surrendered. You know those real deep cries where you just feel your body let go and you let love in, tears streaming for what feels like days...I dislike the definition 'ugly cry' because those are the good ones where there's legit snot everywhere, and you either want to hide or get a hug. In the year approaching explant, I had more release sessions like this than any year of my life. Later I learned, it was these purges that lead me to my purpose.

I began my research for the millions of women who are in the dark about this. I stayed up until 1, 2, 3 a.m., sifting through the studies, the stories of suffering.

I stand up every day as a group administrator to support tens of thousands of women in Breast Implant Illness forums. Women who are often lost, scared and confused... Feeling deceived because they didn't know all these things before they said *yes* to implants. Why? Well, because surgeons are not legally obligated to tell them.

There have been *zero* long-term studies to support the safety of implants…and I'm not ok with this, and neither are the women who were also deceived. Apparently, in the beginning, our voices weren't loud enough. Now, they are. The FDA is finally listening after *decades* of woman warriors speaking up about how their implants made them sick and nearly killed them. Some weren't so fortunate. A dear personal friend's mother died because of her breast implants. So, this "Rise Up" call is for her too!

Implants are toxic to all of us! The UK knows this… And most countries have actually *banned* implants. Many are even *funding* women to have them removed. But why not in the USA? If you haven't yet discovered for yourself, America spends more on *healthcare* than any other industrialized country in the world-- but ranks nearly dead last in overall *health*.

This book about breast implants and what they represent to me is: freedom, starting with examining where we lost it, giving our power away to trusting these governing body's to 'look out for our health'. For nearly a century, it's been prescriptions and procedures over people. Our inclination towards cosmetic surgery and perfection trumps our natural individuality at the behest of our health, overriding all notions of body positivity. The tides are turning fast. We're waking up and we're demanding answers. Who is watching out for *our* well-being? Who is protecting *us*?

The continued widespread idealization of breast implants, despite a lack of long-term research to prove their safety, is on par to become one of the biggest FDA cover-ups in history; and I want to help put it on the map by presenting you with the research I compiled over the course of the past year and a half.

Once I came to the realization that I am here on a mission to ascend this flawed humanity in order to assist universal healing, I was able to accept, forgive and love myself just the way I am. Rather than seeing myself as a broken failure, I am inclined to see my suffering as a gift—one which would reveal such profound truths that it could achieve an undeniably significant transformation. I have been exactly where you are now. I have walked in Emily's shoes, and NOW I am here to help!

If Emily's story resonates with you, I want you to know you are not going crazy, I see you and understand your suffering. I want to tell you about the top four implications of Breast Implant Illness - Toxicity, Infection, Trauma and Shame (yes, it would be a funny abbreviation if it weren't for the suffering it causes) -- as well as proven solutions to reverse it. So, let's start with my experience.

Chapter 2: My Story

I never even considered undergoing plastic surgery. Until, in 2009, I moved to Orange County, the breast implant and plastic surgery capital of the world. As my friends say, the "land of pristine beaches and fake beeches."

In 2010, I began bodybuilding and started competing in bikini competitions. I lost a lot of body fat, my chest looked flat, and I needed to fix it, *stat*. (Remember, laser-focused when it comes to looks).

At the end of 2010, when I modeled for my very first photo shoot, I was unabashedly told, "You'll never get your pro card and get on the cover of *Oxygen Magazine*-- unless you get DD's. All the girls have them." I was so pissed at the photographer, but... I started looking around... And, he was right. It was the exception to *not* have implants in the bodybuilding industry. Within weeks, I felt the pressure to conform.

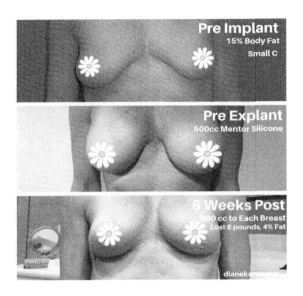

The many masks of my breasts

Around that same time, I did my second bikini competition and won First Overall. If I could qualify for nationals *without* boobs, imagine what I would achieve *with* them. My competitor friends pretty much all had them, so I went shopping for boobs.

With my "whatever it takes to *win*" mentality, and flashbacks to my 8-year-old self playing with Barbie dolls, with the engrained belief that big boobs = beauty, I found a great surgeon and bought myself some DD's 500CC Allergan Silicone implants, under the muscle, for Christmas of 2011. Yay me, I got some D's. I felt so hot…. you remember that feeling?

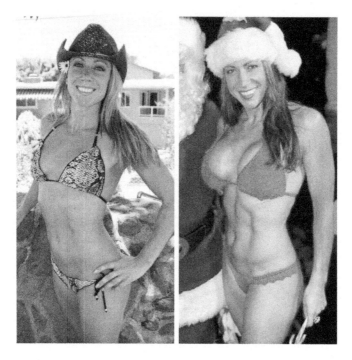

Me without implants summer 2011, then 5 months later with big bazookas

Since I had a week of recovery, I decided it would be a good idea to have all of the silver amalgam teeth fillings that I accumulated since I was a little girl, replaced with porcelain at the same time. At the time, I wanted them replaced more for aesthetic reasons than out of concern for my health. Holistic and biological dentists are the only qualified doctors who are trained and equipped to remove them safely, considering the high levels of mercury vapor released during removal, but I did it the cheap way, which did not come with that level of protection. Little did I know how *stupid* of an idea that was (palm to forehead, *please* do not repeat this mistake). I had no idea what I know now, which you will learn in this book, that I should have been preparing pre and post silver filling removal, how to chelate mercury so it didn't get reabsorbed into my body. For two months I was on top of the world, until my medications wore off....

All of a sudden, I started to look like I was six months pregnant. I had massive stomach pains that felt like a small Ninja was living in my small intestines, constantly poking at me with her sword. I began to refer to my stomach as bipolar bowels, taking turns from constipation to diarrhea. It was a literal shit show. Maybe it was all of the bodybuilding supplements with their high sugar alcohols and artificial sweeteners, ingredients? I had no idea, but I brought these incessant qualms to my show coach trainer. He said, "You're probably just really carbohydrate sensitive, we need to decrease them and increase your protein intake."

Two weeks later, one week before my "Best in California" competition, I looked leaner than ever, but also felt worse than ever. I was lightheaded, nearly passing out, and scared AF.

I stepped on stage for my show and felt 'off'. There I was standing on stage, abs exposed, with the worst gas in the world. You know how bad gas feels when you're alone, compound that when you're nearly naked, with bright lights blasted on your whole body, front and center, ten judges picking you apart with their scratch pads, commanding "Quarter turn to the right." I was feeling awful and awkward. I didn't feel myself and although my trainers said I had looked the best I ever had, and would do really well, I took eleventh, out of 14. How did this happen? I thought I was *ready*. I walked off stage with my heart sunk into my clear bikini heels and was then met with a barrage of insulting comments from my coach.

He accused me of being a complete disaster on stage. My other coach agreed with intense anger, and told me how embarrassed I made him, how it would impact his reputation in the industry. It was my first show with my new implants. Was it because of that? Did my higher self-know better, as if I had somehow betrayed my body. Did I win the shows before and do so well, so fast, because I was being true to *myself*, rather than an industry? I felt owned, controlled, imprisoned. How did I get here? That reflection and introspection landed me in a dark depression for weeks...

After my embarrassing loss, I took to my bed for a week, shut the curtains, laid in darkness, and ate "normal people" food. My weight increased ten pounds, from 135 to 145, overnight. I felt... Lost. I invested so much time, hope, energy and money with an intention to *win*. In one year, I had spent over $25,000: on my bikini ($2,500), buying boobs ($8,000), bodybuilding shows ($800 per show), trainers ($800 per month), and posing coaches ($500 per show), and that didn't even take into consideration what I was spending on supplements ($600 per month) as well as about $500 per month on dangerous drugs that were and still are standard in the "industry" which might as well be called "Instagram." I know this for a fact because I have helped a lot of women on the other side of competing. Heroin, meth, cocaine, HGH, Clenbuterol, diuretics, phentermine, steroids; I've seen it *all*. So, once breast implants were added to that toxic mess of chemicals, mercury, along with scarfing down six meals a day, I hit a wall. I officially lost myself and consequently embarked on a quest to shape my new identity.

I share all of this with you because we have such a skewed perception of what it truly means to be healthy, happy and fit. When I started competing, I had more friends, fans and followers reaching out to ask for help than ever before. I couldn't keep up with it. My business skyrocketed, I was showered with compliments, and got paid to be a fitness model-- all the while feeling like a *huge* hypocrite on the inside. If my main goal was to be InstaFamous by doing squat videos and teaching people how to meal prep while flaunting my cleavage, as an Influencer, I would have made millions by now. But my soul wasn't in it, and I sure as hell wasn't ready to sell my soul to the lies of the fitness industry.

Sure, I worked hard, as I always had... I played soccer my whole life and even played professionally at the highest level in the WPSL in the USA and the Bundesliga in Germany, but I never once "cheated" in so many ways as I did then. People *thought* it was just "diet and exercise" -- eat more frequent meals, eat less calories overall, exercise more, get the most popular whey protein, drink casein at night and take a shit load of supplements. Ugh... Dear thirty-year-old Diane, I'm sorry I put you through all of that... *But...* It was all necessary, so I would ultimately discover the

39

consequences, discern what *not* to do and finally share everything I've uncovered, in this book, ten years later.

Soon after, when my depression lifted, I was ready to act. So, I moved to Hollywood with my then boyfriend, who was building a film studio. Both of us worked twelve plus hours per day. At that time, I became certified as a personal trainer and sports nutritionist, but something was still missing. I felt an inner yearning to get in deeper touch with my true self. So, I eventually enrolled as a yoga teacher trainee. I thought *that* would be *it*. I would find my happy if I did more yoga and taught it to others. I had already been practicing yoga for ten years, so this seemed like the next best "enlightened" thing to do.

During my training, I felt the *worst* back pain in my whole life. My updogs were more like flat dogs and I suddenly noticed how much my boobs were getting in the way of pretty much every pose I attempted. Handstands were *hard* and I always felt off center, top heavy, struggling to "hold myself up." My shoulders, neck and back all began to take the hit and it felt like I was getting old, fast.

After a year of this, in 2012, I decided to travel the world solo. During this time, my health deteriorated even more. I got *really* sick in India and had my first experience with recurrent ear infections that wouldn't quit, even with the strongest of Ayurvedic medications. I still hadn't attributed anything to my breast implants.

It was in 2013 when it all started changing for me. I returned from my world travels and enrolled to become a functional diagnostic nutrition practitioner. I had heard great things about using advanced labs and protocols to help people heal from the root causes of whatever they were struggling with. When I got my labs back, I was in shock. To this day I still am one of the most difficult cases I've seen.

My hormones were "off." I had estrogen dominance and was definitely suffering the symptoms of it. I had high cortisol and low melatonin at night, which is what I refer to as a reverse curve-- when your sleep hormones dip and your stress hormones simultaneously rise.. This causes that feeling of "wired and tired" so you're physically exhausted, yet your mind is racing, and your sleep is therefore compromised. Both of these hormones help to keep inflammation in check, so clearly, my body was working overtime to clear *something* out of my body.

I ran a food sensitivity panel on myself and learned that coffee, polysorbate 80, bananas, and several other "healthy foods" didn't agree with me. I was frustrated because even though I was eating healthy, several of my favorite foods were on the list. I carefully cut them out and then once I stopped drinking coffee, I finally noticed my first shift-- accomplishing some *major* belly bloat reduction.

However, my tests also showed that my immune system was on high alert, producing higher levels of something called Secretory IgA, the gold standard immune defense marker. When I do labs on my clients, I examine to assess how well their body is mounting protection to chemicals, bad bugs, food reactions, etc.

I had off the chart levels of all pathogens-- candida/fungal overgrowth, opportunistic (toxic) bacteria and also Small Intestine Bacterial Overgrowth, (a.k.a. SIBO). My first test showed no parasites, but more on that later because they eventually showed up... And never left, no matter how many cleanses I did.

I had a *super* low metabolism, that is to say slow bowel motility, poor digestive capacity, and a sluggish thyroid, determined by my mineral levels and ratios. And considering how backed up my elimination pathways were, I had dangerously high levels of heavy metal toxicity-- lead, copper, mercury, cadmium, aluminum and more. At first, I thought it was my birth control because one of my mentors, Dr. Rick Malter, discovered high levels of copper on that first hair tissue mineral analysis. And at the time I had a copper IUD. After months of researching the effects of copper toxicity, I began to recognize how closely they aligned with my symptoms. Running up the hill was more strenuous than it was two years before I had *both* implants and the IUD. But at that time, no one was talking about Breast Implant Illness. However, birth control was a hot topic-- believed by many to be a root cause for toxicity as well as digestive and hormonal chaos. I decided to remove my IUD (2014), which was met with resistance from my OB-GYN doctor who said, "But it's perfectly in place and your blood tests are fine, why would you remove it?" It was my first experience standing up

42

for myself, when I politely replied, "Because I know it's not good for me and, in fact, I think it's poisoning me."

Yet, once I removed my birth control... I felt better for a while... Until I hit another wall. I self-ran my first fully comprehensive thyroid lab, which revealed high antibodies to my thyroid. Clinically, this would be diagnosed as Hashimoto's Hypothyroid.

All of my systems were in SOS mode. So, I tried responding to my body's "mayday" by detoxing.

In 2016, my skin rashes began. They were so painful, I had to go to the Urgent Care, since everything I had tried didn't work: essential oils, topical ointments, supplements-- even OTC allergy meds did nothing. The doctors biopsied the rashes and found candida on my chest as well as bacterial overgrowth on my armpits. Both were so bad I had cystic-looking acne on my chest and neck, as well as golf ball sized pocket filled rashes on my armpits. I scratched until I bled. I was literally uncomfortable in my own skin. I was constantly in tears and couldn't even sleep.

It was around this time, I got an email from my friend and detox author/expert Anna Rodgers who had written an article on Breast Implants: the ticking time bomb. I read it, but I wasn't ready to absorb it, nor admit that it might be my implants. After all, I loved them, and they felt "fine", so I figured, "It must be something that just happens to *some* women." A month later, my friend and fellow FDN practitioner and detox expert, Wendy Myers, messaged me and told me she was getting hers removed. I thought, "Wow that sucks, aren't you afraid you're going to look weird with your boobs all deflated?" She got a great surgeon and blogged about it, but I had no interest in reading. My head was still under the sand. If *only* I listened to my intuition, *then*... It would have saved me tens of thousands of dollars, and more...

In December of 2016, I was at my worst. I had pills in my hand and I wanted to end it. My friend, Barry Selby talked me off the ledge and I went into another week of depression. It was Christmas, but I wasn't filled with joy. I wanted to hide. I felt alone in my fight. I felt like I had tried everything. I tried more and more different approaches, but the situation with my rashes, parasites and infections just kept getting worse. I even did the thing I thought I would *never* do and went to the urgent care where they prescribed Prednisone, which turns off your immune system, so it can no longer react to the chemicals, pathogens and toxic waste in your body, thus eliminating the symptoms. But it does *not* get to the root of why you have the symptoms because it does not remove the things your body is reacting to. After years of trying to detox said chemicals, pathogens and toxic waste, I was desperate. I was pissed at myself for dying my hair pink the year before. I should have known better. But that *still* didn't work.

Fast-forward one year; in a last-ditch effort to illuminate my spinal issues, I elected to try a Thermogram. At the time, my back was really hurting. I have had back problems since I was 18, but after 20 years of various therapies (consistent chiropractic adjustments every year, $25k+ on spinal decompression treatments, acupuncture etc.), I was on a mission to resolve my back issues once and for all. What I found baffled me! There were little lumps in the scan around my right breast and the inflammation around my back lit up deep red like a wildfire, without a single firefighter in sight to put it out.

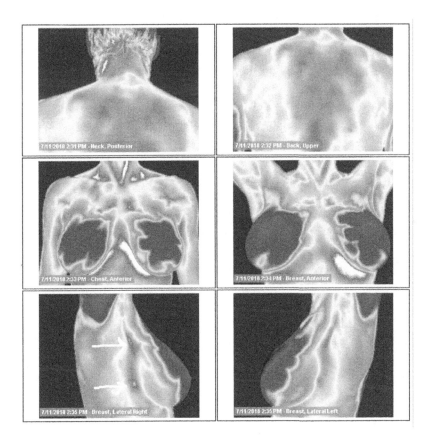

In a thermogram, red means inflammation and not good. See the lumps in my right breast?

It was after this discovery that my mind *finally* opened to the possibility that I might have what my friend Anna referred to as Breast Implant Illness, two years prior. So, I began my research, did *more* labs, and what I found was this:

- I *still* had parasites-- more organisms and an increased diversity of species
- My bacterial load had increased
- I scored super high on my mold test
- My mineral levels coded me for high likelihood of depression, fatigue and gastritis
- I had high copper toxicity yet was deficient on the cellular level. This means copper can't actually get into the cell, usually because it is blocked by toxicity, such as heavy metals. Copper is an important mineral for beauty and it prevents gray hair.

I had high estrogen and extremely low progesterone, a condition known as estrogen dominance... *Still*, five years after running my first functional lab in 2013, and consistently doing *a ton* of work trying to correct it, such as hoarding broccoli, supplementing with DIM and CDG (known to flush excess estrogen), changed birth control, stopped using birth control all together, and reduced my exposure to estrogen mimicking toxins like plastic, pesticides, petroleum-based beauty products and more.

This time I had barely detectable levels of testosterone, low melatonin and completely flat-lined cortisol. No wonder I was tired, my body could no longer make stress hormones to give me energy.

What was confusing was that I had won a bikini competition around this time, and the way I prepped for it was by simply giving my body more detox, protein and compound muscle building exercises. I was able to get down to 14 percent body fat. I looked my best ever, not emaciated nor excessively buff, yet on the inside I was still *super* sick, according to my labs. So that's what is so confusing: A fit appearance on the outside does not equal a healthy inside. And that is the case with so many women who have BII, since the majority of us are more concerned with looking good, and what I have noticed is a 'perfectionist' mentality. Here's what I looked like on the inside, and I was starting to really break down. I knew I had to do something…and soon!

Breast Implant Illness Symptoms
Diane Kazer

Insomnia or Low Melatonin
Low ATP Production
High Homocysteine
High Heavy Metals on Hair & Urine labs
Estrogen Dominance Symptoms
MTHFR gene
Chemical sensitivity
Food Intolerances
Belly Bloat or SIBO Diagnosis
Leaky Gut
Lyme Symptoms or Diagnosis
Chronic Viral Infections - HPV, HSV, EBV
Mold like Symptoms
Little to no relief with Chiropractic, PT, massage
Autoimmune Symptoms or diagnosis
Fibromyalgia like symptoms
Thyroid and Adrenal Imbalances
Irritable Bowel or bladder
UTI's & Interstitial Cystitis Diagnosis
Sciatica
Back Pain
Irritability
Intolerance to a$$ holes ;)
Nipple Sensitivity to Cold
Cold hands & Feet
Poor Circulation
Shoulder / Neck Pain
Anxiety
Morning Fatigue & Coffee stops working
Joint Pain
Muscle Pain
Muscle Weakness
Poor Immune function - sick often
Shyness, Apathy, lack of Confidence

Skin Rashes
Body Itching
Chronic Candida
Yeast Infections
Leukoplakia (inner mouth film)
Inflammation
Visual disturbance / Eye Floaters
Lymph swelling and Tenderness
Headaches
Depression
Decreased Libido
Mood swings
Sharp pains around & under breast
Heart palpitations
Difficulty Breathing
Weight Gain
Chronic Fatigue symptoms
Eye lid & face swelling
Night Sweats
Excess Mucous production & excretion
Sensitivity to Electronic Devices
Zaps using Phone, Computer, ipads
Difficulty Concentrating
Memory Loss
Dizzy Standing up
Low Body Temperature
Chills
Temperature Intolerance
Sensitivity to light
Sensitivity to Sound
Hair Loss or Poor Hair growth
Dry skin / hair
Sinus Infections
Recurrent Illness

dianekazer.com

I began my search for a good explant doctor in December of 2018. After interviewing eleven different doctors, I finally found my surgeon in Newport Beach, CA: Dr. Jon Bradley Strawn. I spoke to him in January and booked it for five months later. What I learned quickly is that it's important to work with a surgeon who specializes in safe and effective explant surgery-- and when you find one, they usually have a waiting list. Fair enough-- I wanted to do it right the first time. After all, my health is my #1 asset and in the past 3 years, feeling it deteriorate was a costly wake up call. In the meantime, I did everything in my power, and spent every minute of my day researching BII: what it was, how we got here, why the FDA allowed it, talking to other women about their experiences, how to prepare for surgery, critical steps to detox, and how to heal post explant.

For five months, my symptoms got worse and many more of the ones listed here surfaced toward the end. My cold fingers and toes were so unbearable I couldn't type but for ten minutes at a time. The sharp pains across my chest and electro-shocks became more frequent and scarier. My sensitivity to stimulation was at an all-time high, to the point that I stayed home away from crowds to avoid any noise pollution, artificial scents, high energy and other unnecessary stressors. The scariest thing to me was the difficulty I had breathing. I was lucky if I got *one* good deep breath in all day. I was beginning to mourn the person I once was and felt as though I would do anything to get me back. I even lost interest in exercise, as it was

48

painful, I was exhausted after and it took a longer time to recover. And ugh…I was 15 pounds heavier than my usual healthy weight. The last time that happened was in college when I was a server at a pub in London, but that's because I was drinking lots of Guinness and living it up.

It was maddening to feel me quickly slip away, and what infuriated me most was the FDA. Why would they approve implants in the first place? With every woman's story, all the suffering, the lack of data; the presence of data later to be burned, never to be published; the dismissal of critical reports of symptoms and side effects; the skewed results-- and then discovering all of the science that came out in December of 2018 with over 100,000 women, the largest study on women with breast implants that revealed higher incidence of stillbirths, auto immune disease, depression, suicide and pathogenic overload, such as bacteria and Candida. When I read what you are about to read in this book, I dove head first into investing all of my efforts to understand the impact of having breast implants inside our sacred temples. Who is most effected? How do we reclaim our health? Is it even possible to do this, while also retaining our beautiful breasts? I made it my mission to help other women going through the same trauma so that they don't have to suffer like I did. From suffering to sovereignty, I turned my pain into my purpose.

What you are about to acquire in this book is the *fast track* path to healing. I took these same steps to prepare for explant, through recovery and even now, one year later. I will spare you about 90 percent of what didn't work so you can go straight to what does. I will teach you how to customize your path and, if you so choose, enlist the support of practitioners, programs and products that are worth investing toward-- increasing your odds of getting better, faster. I explanted on May 31, 2019, and it's been a wild ride since— one full of many beautiful lessons.

My hope is that you will learn from my errors, so you don't have to repeat the mistakes I made yourself. If that sounds like music to your tits, then promise me this: you'll pass it on to other women suffering in silence, to those who seek self-love over silicone!

Chapter 3: What Is Breast Implant Illness?

Here is the most dangerous *myth* women with implants carry in their mind:

- Myth: My breast implants don't cause me any problems. My boobs look and feel fine.

- Truth: Illness caused by implants are a conglomerate of eighty plus symptoms and diagnoses, such as brain fog, depression/anxiety, skin issues, hair loss, weight gain, pain, inflammation, chronic fatigue, auto immune disease, frequent sicknesses, gut problems, low body temp/blood pressure, infertility and more! They impact every woman's health and the evidence of that lies in the capsule that our immune system forms around the implant, essentially walling it off from the body.

Here is a complete list of toxins in breast implants:

38 TOXINS IN BREAST IMPLANTS
XenoEstrogens, Metals, Plastic,etc

1 - Methyl ethyl ketone (neurotoxin)
2 - Cyclohexanone (neurotoxin)
3 - Isopropyl Alcohol
4 - Denatured Alcohol
5 - Acetone (neurotoxin used in nail polish remover)
6 - Urethane
7 - Polyvinyl chloride (neurotoxin)
8 - Amine
9 - Toulene
10 - Dicholormethane (carcinogen)
11 - Chloromethane
12 - Ethyl acetate (neurotoxin)
13 - Silicone
14 - Sodium fluoride
15 - Lead Based Solder
16 - Formaldehyde
17 - Talcum powder
18 - Platinium
19 - Silica + (2)

20 - Oakite (cleaning solvent)
21 - Methyl 2 Cynanoacrylates
22 - Ethylene Oxide (Carcinogen)
23 - Xylene (neurotoxin)
24 - Hexon
25 - 2-Hedanone
26 - Thixon-OSN-2
27 - Stearic Acid
28 - Zinc Oxide
29 - Naptha (rubber solvent)
30 - Phenol (neurotoxin)
31 - Benzene (carcinogen/neurotoxin)
32 - Lacquer thinner
33 - Epoxy resin
34 - Epoxy hardener
35 - Printing ink
36 - Metal cleaning acid
37 - Colour pigments as release agents
38 - Heavy metals such as aluminium (neurotoxin linked to Alzheimer's and auto immune disorders)

"The shell on silicone and saline implants is comprised of silicone and over 40 other toxic chemicals: tin, zinc, cadmium, mercury, arsenic, formaldehyde and talc to name a few. Your immune system is constantly fighting them, leaving you vulnerable to other illnesses."

dianekazer.com

But I thought they were just made of silicone? Nope, turns out they didn't tell us the whole truth. In addition to that, there seem to be women who are at a higher risk for symptoms than others.

Risk factors that increase incidence of BII:

- Poor detox genetics - such as MTHFR

- Body dysmorphia

- An eating disorder or a history of eating disorder

- A mental diagnosis or unstable mood

- Auto immune disease

- A history of cancer

- A predisposition for any of the above risk factors

- Frequent exposure to exceptionally high levels of toxins (such as hairdressers)

- Allergies

- Skin issues

52

- Spinal issues

And here's what to look out for as the most common symptoms of BII:

"How is this happening?" You may ask yourself. "I was assured they were safe and posed no harm." I hear it in the BII communities over and over again.

Apparently, silicone is not inert, as some doctors and implant companies have claimed. It sweats and bleeds from the insertion, which means even if yours do not leak, tear, or rupture, your body still gets poisoned-- and there are studies to prove it.

One study revealed that approximately 74% of women with implants had silicone migration to their lymph nodes. Implants are permeable... Doctors will tell you that nothing can get in or out, but how do they explain the saline implants that are covered in mold on the inside? Or the silicone implants that turn yellow and have speckles of something resembling mold inside them? How did this happen?

Silicone also depletes your body's collagen stores. That's why a lot of women with breast implants suffer from premature aging and joint pain. D4 (also known as octamethylcyclotetrasiloxane from silicone) has a proven impact on levels of LH and FSH— hormones required for ovulation. This points to why many women report irregular periods, infertility and early menopause, some as early as in their mid-twenties.

33 Ways Breast Implants Destroy Your Body

Would you have chosen implants if your doctor handed you this list?

1. Increased risk for cancer:

Breast implants can cause cancer of the immune system, called anaplastic large-cell lymphoma (ALCL), which is a rare type of blood cancer. So far, it has been detected in 457 women with breast implants. Interestingly, removing the implants usually eliminates the disease, but some women have opted for chemotherapy, and seventeen deaths from the cancer have been reported worldwide. What are symptoms of BIA-ALCL? The most common is excessive fluid buildup around the breast implant, which can cause pain, swelling or lumps in the breast or armpit.

2. Increased risk of other cancers:

A second NCI study found a 21% overall increased risk of cancer for women with implants, compared with women of the same age in the general population. The increase was primarily due to an increase in brain cancer, respiratory tract cancers, cervical cancer and vulvar cancer.

3. Increased risk for suicide:

Women who have breast implants are *three* times more likely to commit suicide than women in the general population.

4. Increased risk for depression:

A Danish study, funded by implant manufacturer Dow Corning, found an increase in depression among women with implants and a *five* to *seven* times higher chance of taking antidepressants than women without implants.

5. They destroy your immune system:

Because your body is trying to "push out" and attack anything "that it detects as non-self" your immune system gets tired and eventually, your immune system fails because it's overwhelmed. Think your typical Monday, only ten times worse, *and* it's Monday inside your body *everyday*.

When the immune system is impaired, your defenses are *down*. This allows various infections in the body to grow and thrive, causing symptoms that replicate the common cold, flu, allergy or who knows what— you just feel tired and don't know why.

6. They are hormone disruptors:

Have you heard of a class of toxins known as xeno-estrogens? It simply means "foreign toxin that acts like estrogen in the body." Plastics are a big one. Silicone is another. These chemicals impair your fragile endocrine gland system, or your TAO (thyroid/adrenals/ovaries). As long as those glands aren't optimal, you'll find yourself with hormone deficiencies and imbalances that just might lend themselves to endometriosis, PCOS, thyroid disease, chronic exhaustion, adrenal fatigue, fibrocystic breasts (painful lumps around your breasts) PMS, PMDD and more... And no amount of medication *really* does the trick. I'll walk you more through in the 'labs' chapter.

7. They increase the stress hormone cortisol, depleting the adrenal and thyroid glands:

When the body perceives a "foreign" object, the adrenals release, cortisol to put out the fire of inflammation. When this is happening twenty-four/seven, eventually the adrenals cannot withstand the permanent wildfire within. The fire therefore spreads-- thus the inflammation cannot be fought, so it goes unaddressed. And we go round and round...

8. Sex hormones decrease in many women:

When the stress hormones rise, sex and sleep hormones decrease because the body prioritizes cortisol as a fight-or-flight response. Wondering where your sex drive went? Your ability to build muscle? Burn fat? Your testosterone is probably shot like mine was. What about Vaginal Dryness? Depression? Infertility?

Estrogen and progesterone are on "vaycay", and unfortunately this is where hormone replacement therapy and bioidenticals simply don't stand a chance. They'll stop working too because they're but mere Band-Aids, unable to resolve the root cause of your hormonal issues.

9. They dirty our genes:

Have you ever had a 23andMe done? Been tested for BRCA? How about MTHFR gene mutation? What you may have heard is that "You can't do anything about your genes, you're stuck with them." This is true. *But* what's left unsaid is you can actually turn off your bad genes and turn on your *good* genes simply by nourishing your body, cleaning up your lifestyle and up-leveling your mindset. It's called epi-genetics-- but none of that applies when you have implants, because they turn "on" our genetic mutations so that the "bad genes" can act out. Look at what runs in your family. Implants likely increase your odds of those conditions. Until they're removed, implants will continue to tempt underlying genetic disadvantages due to the incessant, permanent stress they present. Those with MTHFR issues, (I'm double homozygous-- double screwed), in my opinion, should stay far away from implants because we tend to lack the ability to detox efficiently.

10. Implants are full of heavy metals:

Implants disrupt mineral levels in the body since they occupy the same receptor sites on cells. As long as metals are blocking these receptors, minerals can't get in, and since hormones need minerals for production, hormone levels are eventually impaired. Additionally, the body will store these metals in the safest zones, such as fat cells, which guess what? The brain is 60 percent fat... Hence why it can feel like your brain just isn't working right, and... Wait, what article am I writing? Oh, sorry... Just some brain inflammation there for a moment!

11. Inflammation increases:

Inflammation is the root cause of 95% of disease today. If you've struggled to lose weight and you have implants, perhaps you are experiencing inflammation coupled with fat expansion, as your body stores the toxins bleeding from your implants. I've seen *so many* women literally diet, cleanse and exercise program hop with no success... Until, one day, they finally explant and lose ten pounds in one week, twenty in a month... I had no idea I had 15 pounds of inflammation to lose, until I explanted.

12. You may lose your health insurance:

In some states, major health insurance providers have refused to insure women with breast implants. Some insurers have sold health insurance to women with implants, but charged them more. While some insurers refuse to cover specific illnesses contracted by female patients with breast implants, others refuse to cover any problems in the breast area whatsoever. Furthermore, it did not matter if a particular disease was related to implants, if the patient was diagnosed with a disease, she would automatically be excluded from coverage.

13. Implants reduce detection of breast cancer:

Implants can interfere with the detection of breast cancer in mammograms. Approximately 55% of breast tumors can hide under the implant. This statistic is unrelated to the increased risk of rupture.

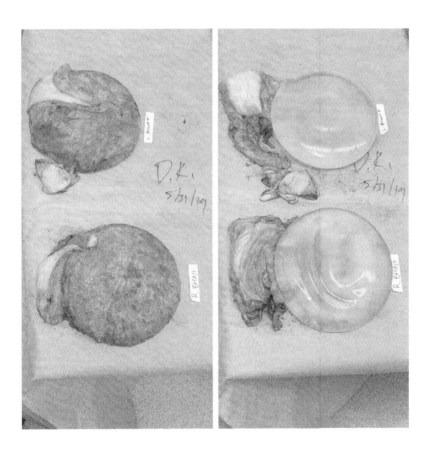

These are my breast implants with a hamburger looking capsule surrounding it. This tissue is created by our highly intelligent body that 'builds a wall' around the implants to protect it from exposure to toxins and non-self-parts. It's vital you work with an explant surgeon who knows how to properly remove this capsule via an en-bloc procedure.

14. They increase risk of auto-immune disease:

All implants are "foreign objects," and a woman's body reacts to the foreign object by forming a capsule of scar tissue around the implant itself (as shown in picture above, taken post explant surgery). As a study sampling over 100,000 women concluded, "The risk of certain autoimmune diseases increased by 800% (Sjogren Syndrome), 700% (scleroderma), and 600% (arthritis) for women with implants compared to the general population of women of the same age and demographics."

15. Implants are linked to fibromyalgia:

A study conducted by FDA scientists found a statistically significant link between implants and fibromyalgia, as well as several other connective tissue diseases. The study focused on women who had silicone breast implants for at least six years and found that women with leaking silicone implants were significantly more likely to report a diagnosis of painful and debilitating diseases such as fibromyalgia, dermatomyositis, polymyositis, Hashimoto's thyroiditis, mixed connective tissue disease, pulmonary fibrosis, eosinophilic fasciitis, and polymyalgia.

16. Implants are linked to rheumatologic disease:

A study by Aziz et al. examined 95 women who had silicone gel-filled breast implants and rheumatological symptoms. These researchers found that the symptoms improved in forty-two of the forty-three women who had their breast implants removed (97%), as oppose to replaced. In contrast, rheumatological symptoms worsened in fifty of the fifty-two women who did not have their implants removed (96%).

17. You are at higher odds to lose your baby:

Stillbirths increased by 450% in gestating women with implants. Stillbirth is when a baby dies in the womb after twenty weeks of pregnancy.

18. Implant chemicals can be passed through breastfeeding:

According to the Institute of Medicine (IOM), women with any kind of breast surgery, including breast implant surgery, are at least *three* times as likely to have an inadequate milk supply for breastfeeding. Concerns about the safety of breast milk have also been raised, but there has not been enough research to resolve this issue.

19. Bacteria and mold grow in and around them, in between the implants and the implant shell, aka capsule

Bacteria or mold can grow in saline implants. Doctors have expressed concerns about the bacteria or mold being released into the body if the implant breaks. In my practice, we've consistently seen women with mold symptoms that mimic candida, but they can't figure out where it's coming from. Light bulb moment?

20. They cause chronic candidiasis:

Ever wondered why that candida diet didn't stick? Or why you have a hard time saying no to sugar, carbs, and caffeine? Implants hire your immune system to work a full-time job, in order to detox upwards of thirty different leaching chemicals-- which over time, causes the immune system to wear out. Once that happens, it has a harder time fighting off pathogens like candida, superbugs and many other toxins. Brain fog, itchiness, rashes and hair loss anyone?

21. 50-75% have major complications within three years:

The FDA found that most implant patients have at least one serious complication within three years after getting silicone or saline implants. Studies of saline breast implants and silicone gel breast implants conducted by implant manufacturers have shown that within the *first three* years, approximately three out of four reconstruction (breast cancer) patients (75%) and almost half (50%) of first-time augmentation patients experienced at least one local complication-- such as pain, infection, hardening, or they necessitate additional surgery.

22. They all break:

Eventually. In a study conducted by FDA scientists, most women had at least one broken implant within eleven years, while the likelihood of rupture increases every year thereafter.

23. There are no real studies proving their safety:

When they approved silicone gel breast implants in 2006, the FDA required two implant manufacturers, Allergan and Mentor, to each conduct ten-year studies of at least 40,000 women to determine why implants break, how long they're expected to last, and what the longer-term health consequences of broken or leaking breast implants might be. Those studies were never completed, nor did the

FDA require Allergan or Mentor to substitute its initial demands with similarly well-designed studies.

24. The studies are skewed:

In late 2005, the FDA requested a ten-year study of 40,000 women with Inamed (Allergan) or Mentor (Johnson & Johnson) breast implants. Several women testified that they were thrown out of the implant studies when they decided to remove their implants or if they reported serious health problems from their breast implants. One Mentor employee admitted that executives ordered him to destroy documents related to a high rupture rate of Mentor implants. This raises questions about the accuracy of the data presented. Nevertheless, the FDA accepted the studies and maintained that silicone implants were safe and effective (face to palm).

25. They can contribute to leaky gut and cause food sensitivities

Along with allergies, electro-sensitivities and chemical intolerances. When your gut isn't happy, you're not happy. Every symptom leads back to a gut issue, and the toxins from implants destroy our digestive tracks in many ways. Have you noticed, all of a sudden, you're allergic to more foods? Is your body more sensitive to smells? Are you reacting to cosmetics, personal care and beauty products that you didn't react to before? Or possibly even worse, does your partner suddenly reek?

26. They are expensive and inconvenient:

When the FDA approved silicone gel breast implants in November 2006, it stated that women should have a breast MRI three years after getting silicone implants and every two years after that. The purpose of the MRIs is to determine if the silicone gel breast implants are ruptured or leaking, because there are often no symptoms, when they are. Breast MRIs usually cost at least $2,000, and at some facilities they cost more than $5,000. It is important to remove silicone implants if they are ruptured, to avoid the silicone leaking into the breast or lymph nodes. That is an additional expense of at least $5,000 and can be $10,000 or more. Doing the math is certainly important, since 55% of Americans are living paycheck-to-paycheck and many women cannot afford the long-term costs of maintaining this particular cosmetic surgery.

27. They are heavy:

Every 100cc of silicone implant weighs 0.23lbs. Every 100cc of saline implant weighs 0.21lbs. So, a typical 300cc silicone implant weighs 0.69 pounds and a pair of them together weighs 1.38 pounds. 300cc saline implants weigh 0.63lb each or 1.26lbs for both of them. Essentially implants weigh about the same as an equal amount of what breast tissue would weigh. I had 475cc's, which for me, means just over one pound each! Imagine putting a two-pound dumbbell on your chest and having to carry that around with you everywhere you go.

28. They restrict blood flow

To other areas within the body, mainly extremities such as fingers, toes and nipples, which in its extreme form can result in a condition known as Reynaud's. I, myself, have this. White fingertips, cold toes that the thickest socks and gloves won't even warm me up. Talk about inconvenient when you need to type all day.

29. They cause major skin issues and UTI's

For many of us, what the immune system is fighting so hard to protect us from, reject, and detox, is the implants. A biofilm that grows on the surface of the implant, found on the pathology report of every woman who explants, known as Propionibacterium acnes (P. Acnes), can cause a persistent inflammation of surrounding tissue. This leads to the formation of capsular fibrosis, causing acne to proliferate all over the body, which usually does not resolve with antibiotics, because medication cannot penetrate the capsule around the implant, precisely where this bacteria hides, shielded until explant.

30. They can leak silicone into lymph nodes:

Numerous studies have shown silicone leaks into the scar capsules surrounding breast implants, even for implants that are not ruptured. More worrisome, researchers at Case Western Reserve and the Armed Forces Institute of Pathology reported finding silicone in the lymph nodes, which can then migrate to other organs. Once in the body, it is very difficult to detox, and may never fully be cleared from the body.

31. They misalign your spine and ribs:

One study concluded that increased breast weight causes several spinal, postural alterations that reduce the ability to perform dynamic tasks requiring stable balance. They found that implants impair the cervical (neck)-postural physiologic balance, plus a significant increase in lumbar (lower back) lordosis (large inward arch). Due to this misalignment, the pectoral muscles (chest muscles) must bear the additional weight, which pulls the shoulders forward. Although it may not pose as much of an issue for women with stronger posterior shoulder and shoulder blade muscles, many women do not practice regular weight or functional movement training. This results in a feeling of strain and tension that no amount of massaging nor chiropractic adjustments will relieve. The pain is a signal of struggle due to weakness. Additionally, ribs migrate, misalign and concave, especially for those women who have had them in the longest. When this happens, it's difficult to take a deep breath, a classic symptom reported by many patients.

32. They damage nerves:

Any surgery on breasts can, and often does, damage nerves and reduce skin sensation. The amount of loss is unpredictable, but the damage cannot be reversed. Over time, women run the risk of diagnosing multiple sclerosis, an auto-immune disease related to nerve damage.

33. Most of the UK has banned them:

Silicone implants were taken off the market in Europe in 2011 because of a tendency to rupture sooner than other implants. What's worse is it was indicated that silicone was not intended for use in the human body but rather was intended for use in mattresses. Public outrage and concern were so strong that several countries, including France, the United Kingdom, Bolivia and Venezuela agreed to pay for implants to be removed, even for augmentation patients. Headline news as of March 2019, reports that thirty-eight countries total, including thirty-three in Europe, have banned them.

Quite the list, right? If you've read this far, I'm curious what you might be thinking right now. If you're like me, you're in shock, and maybe even denial. I was… It took me *three years* before I was willing to admit to myself it was my implants that were a huge source for my health issues.

And you know what? It's okay if you aren't ready to admit that yours might be too. But for the sake of other women out there, regardless of your opinion on this, please share this book with those you know who have implants. It could really save a life. Just sharing this with them at least gives them the respect to decide for themselves.

What we resist persists and for so many women, until we're ready to listen, symptoms and suffering may continue until we simply cannot ignore the signs any longer.

Are there women who will never show symptoms? Sure... But I'm willing to wager that they're in the minority. If you're a woman with any symptom whatsoever, it might just be tied to your implants. Is it worthwhile to gamble on your health? That's up to you.

But you know what?

If you're willing to open your mind up to alternatives to breast implants, there are amazing new procedures that help you explant (remove your implants and the toxic sac around them), lift your breasts *and* shape them fuller through a process called Fat Transfer, where your skilled surgeon of choice (be very picky, I can help you with this process) can remove fat from the thicker areas of your body through Liposuction and deposit it into your breast tissue.

Game changer, right? Once I heard that, it was "Game On" for me! Because I was scared if I removed my implants, my breasts would look strange. New breasts are coming back into the trend zone. I could add this as number 34: We're not show dogs. We're not Barbies. We're Warrior Women who are standing up and standing out with the natural beauty and essence we were gifted with. No judgment if you are a woman with implants *at all.* I was one myself. Nor will I frown upon a decision to take the risk and keep them, as I did, for so long, electing to bump up my detox, while creating an inflammation reduction strategy. All I can hope is that this book plants a seed, that sprouts into a future wisdom branch empowering you to decide for yourself what makes sense for you.

This book is for those who wish to live in the light and put up a fight against the longer-standing toxic trend of "dying to be beautiful".

One last point. One of the common denominators I have observe in my practice. The women who suffer the most, whether it be from breast implants or not, are the ones who are caging themselves with their unresolved trauma. When you cage trauma, you trap toxins. This is where I have found the magic, the sweet spot of success in the approach now known as CHI. In order to break free from both, it starts with healing the feels you've been suppressing and shaming your whole life!

Chapter 4: Pretty Sure It's My Implants, Now What?

Well done, my friend, congratulations on having an open mind. This is not easy to hear and often times can feel like a feast of surreal, with a side of betrayal. You may be wondering how you got here... After all, you were taught that the FDA should be "looking out" for you. So, I celebrate you for expanding your limits beyond disbelief. Truly. Ok, now, here's what's also important: do not sensationalize implants as the sole source for your health issues. While I'm all about getting back to your beautifully unique Goddess temple, High-Fiving any woman who takes the Courageous journey to Explant, I'm also pragmatic and well researched on a toxic trend towards adopting this:

Myth: Breast implants are the reason for *all* my symptoms and explant is going to solve *all* my health problems. All my symptoms are going to miraculously go away after explant.

Truth: There are hundreds of other reasons why women suffer with symptoms of Breast Implant Illness, not caused by their implants. BII is a *piece* of the picture but not the *whole* picture. Generally, many surgeons will tell you that most of their patients experience a 70% reduction in their symptoms after proper explant, but that is not a blanket statement. There are 3 scenarios that take place within 1-3 months post-surgery. You may:

1. Explant, and feel significantly better.

2. Explant, and experience a reduction of symptoms, but not all.

3. Explant, and feel worse.

And of that, even beyond 3 months, for many women, new symptoms arise, and they feel disappointed because they thought they had addressed the culprit behind their crap-tastic laundry list of symptoms. *I am here to level out the logic here and bust the myth that all you need to do is explant.* Too many women I have supported on this journey, have come to me after a year or more post-explant, feeling frustrated that their symptoms returned, or new ones surfaced. My wish for you is that you go into this explant-battlefield with your mindset screwed on right. Explant is Step Number One on your healing journey. Breast implants or not, it's my belief that all of us need to reduce our toxic load and support our detox pathways on a daily basis, a term I coined ABC, which means "Always be Cleansing." Here's why...

You are literally exposed to thousands of toxins on a daily basis: in your morning "beauty" routine, cosmetics, personal care and cleaning products, the food you eat, the water you drink, and the air you breathe. Other assaults to your precious temple include infections as well as pathogens you accumulate from eating out, sushi, uncooked meats, contaminated produce, swapping fluids with others, vaccinations, cohabitating with our beloved pets, a high carbohydrate diet, processed food and sugar (including alcohol).

Also consider Med Spa treatments such as Botox, which is the #1 most toxic substance in the world, a deadly bacteria, society has conditioned us to spend $1,000 + per year—all in the name of, paradoxically, "anti-aging."

We are now hearing of thousands of women suffering from 'Botox Illness' after treatment, and the side effects are debilitating, during the six-plus months it takes to clear the poison out. Unfortunately, some can even suffer from symptoms permanently.

These "bad bugs" are propagated by over-prescribed antibiotics in addition to consuming animals routinely administered antibiotics. While other industrially harvested food contains herbicides ("weed-killer"), known as Glyphosate (aka Round-Up); our culture obsesses on slathering on anti-bacterial soap and spraying bleach products everywhere. We literally sterilize everything, which unfortunately kills the "good bugs" in the process, depleting our immune system and innate defenders.

REAL TALK: The prevalence of toxins and infections, combined with the amount of stress we are under as a culture, adds to your toxic load, exacerbating BII symptoms.

The most empowering step you can take now, is to begin collecting data on what makes up all of the unique parts of you. In order to determine Root Causes for your symptoms, it's imperative to establish a baseline for understanding which bodily systems need the most attention. As you embark on your Cleanse, Heal, Ignite journey to Overcome BII, know that although you *can* do this alone,

I wouldn't recommend it. Riding solo can get confusing and overwhelming. You don't want to give up before you can even connect all the dots to plot your path ahead.

Alongside working with a skilled Explant surgeon, having a strong, reliable coach, serving as your own personal Health Detective, is the single most empowering thing you can do to not only Overcome BII, but also take charge of your life beyond Explant.

It's my belief that we all benefit from having a coach, therapist, health practitioner, *someone* who will help you see your blind spots, what you don't know that you don't know, and help you discover the keys within to heal yourself. Someone who will challenge you and someone who possesses what I call the 3 E's – Empathy, Experience and Education. In other words, one who has been there, done that and mastered the formula to heal fast. There are a lot of great Functional Medicine and Naturopathic practitioners out there, yet what I have found is that working with one who hasn't been through the suffering you've been through, especially BII, will not be able to provide you with the mental, emotional and spiritual support and patience you will need to bring you back to normal and beyond that-- balance, harmony and bad-assery.

When you open yourself up to healing, it's a very personal journey, so it's paramount the person or team you're working with is able to respectfully, authentically and courageously hold space for you and help you heal yourself, until you're strong enough to withstand the ups and downs of purging toxins, healing your tissues and releasing trauma that causes suffering.

One of the greatest ingredients missing in the health space today are authentic leaders who have done their own healing on a holistic level – mentally, emotionally, physically and spiritually – such that they may be able to provide that same level of treatment to their tribe, teaching them to be their OWN best healer by intuitively learning the language of their body and what their symptoms are speaking to them.

While you can definitely work on detox, take bio-identical hormones, clean up your diet or beauty routine, the real transformation happens when you look at all of the things standing in your way of healing, holistically.

1. Someone who has been through what you've been through – empathy

2. Has invested a lot of time helping women from explant to empowerment-- experience

3. Is well educated on the right functional labs to run, beyond blood testing

4. Addresses your whole body to heal, holistically – gut, hormones, neurotransmitters, detox, mindset, emotional trauma, genetics, lifestyle and more.

5. Teaches you how to listen to your body and trust your intuition. This is key. Otherwise, you'll just be told what to do and won't learn the most valuable lesson in this experience.

6. A unique protocol customized to you, your schedule and lifestyle, considering - detox, diet, sleep, mental, emotional and spiritual blocks. If it's a template protocol everyone is doing, it may help but it won't take you across the finish line.

You're probably wondering what labs you might need, what supplements to take, as well as who can help you to order, interpret and create a healing protocol. This is the trickiest part, and one so many people miss, because the only lab most surgeons value is a standard CBC (Complete Blood Count) and CMP (Comprehensive Metabolic Panel), both being blood tests, which are extremely limiting when it comes to what's going on deep inside of your body, tissues and organs— what actually determines the composition of what's flowing through your blood.

This is the major difference between Allopathic/Western medicine and Homeopathic/Eastern medicine. One numbs out symptoms and the other treats the root cause of them. They both have their value, yet what you should be interested in, should revolve around fixing the core of the problem, so you don't have to spin your wheels chasing symptoms. You probably already know this by now, but that $hit gets exhausting, and your adrenals have already been through enough, am I right?

In order to get your "Big Picture" of Health, dive into the all-encompassing health of your tissues, hormones, gut, genetics, immune function and neurotransmitters. Beyond toxicity levels, it's important to consider all of the puzzle pieces that make up your anatomy-- everything that has been affected through this BII journey, and even prior to it. Having this information can set the stage for a rapid recovery and increase the odds of you feeling better than ever, in the fastest time possible. It could also be the magical key to unlocking some major health blocks—ones could make or break your energy and body post explant. I've treated a lot of women after surgery that, had we known the information you're about to learn, could have prevented unwanted chaos and pain as well wasted money, time and energy that could have been spent on preparing their bodies for the explant and ensuring a cascade of healing beyond.

✳ LABS TO GET BEFORE

- Blood and lab work, BIA-ALCL, pathogen reports
- Scans (MRI, ultrasound)
- Thermogram, preferably a SonoCine (instead of a mammogram)

Other labs to consider:

- Urinary Hormone panel
- Thyroid - complete panel (including antibodies, reverse T3, ferritin and more)
- EBV - Full panel including Early Antigens
- Gut panel via stool (inflammation, infections, immune health, imbalances)
- Leaky gut

- Genetics

- Heavy metals and mineral (urine or hair)

- Mold (if suspicious of mold and/or lived/worked in a moldy building)

- Lyme and other special considerations (if Lyme symptoms present)

✳ LABS TO GET AFTER

When you decide to explant, there's a right way and a wrong way to prepare for it, one to help rebuild your body better.

While you certainly can just explant, I *highly* advise against it. For years your body has been harboring plastic, metals and silicone stored deep in the tissues, brain and lymph. All that must be extracted properly.

Then, the gut and hormones need a lot of love too. As does your heart, with lots of self-love and self-care. We're living in *the most* toxic times, with the greatest amount of trauma to contend with, emotionally, spiritually and mentally.

Breast implants or *not*, our bodies need a *Toxin and Trauma Evacuation Plan* so you can connect with your highest self and deliver the mission you were born to serve.

This is the journey that, when taken, works miracles to bring you back to life and beyond.

How Do I Work toward Explant in the Fastest, Most Productive Way Possible?

First off, take a deep, cleansing breath, sister. I am here for you. While this can be a frightening topic, you don't have to do this by yourself, nor do you have to suffer in silence.

A good start is to check your toxic load. Visit my website - dianekazer.com - to take the Neurotoxic Questionnaire. It's a symptom checklist you can take to your doctor/surgeon to communicate your symptoms and goals with them, and track your symptoms from pre to post explant, and beyond through your cleanse, heal, ignite journey. I'll also give you some basic recommendations when you're done.

Beyond that, for *now*, the most important things are:

#1 Listen to the language of your symptoms and give your body what it needs. Surrender, slow down, self-care, self-love, support your tender heart. Ask your body, gently, what it needs, where pain lives, and give to those parts of yourself. I share a lot of options to do this in future Chapters of this book.

#2 Nourish your temple wherever you are in your journey. Start with lymph and liver-loving foods (leafy greens, nuts and seeds, garlic, turmeric, ginger, citrus, berries, beets) rest, hydrate, etc. *Not all* symptoms we experience are from the breast implants. A lot also has to do with what we eat, how we hydrate, move, rest, how we think and talk to ourselves, the chemicals we put on our

bodies and use in our homes, the people we surround ourselves with, and where we spend our time (in nature vs in cubicles, etc.). I cannot stress enough the importance of building a foundation for health by grounding and nourishing your temple, reducing your toxic load, and calming your nervous system.

#3 Research your options: doctors, insurance, labs, procedures, scans, etc. This is an important step, and yet also the most time-consuming. If you don't find someone who knows how to remove the source properly, you are never going to be able to impact your health. This is why it's so important to find a surgeon who has a proven track record of en bloc explant with complete capsulectomy. You can find a list of Expert Explant Surgeons on my website. These are the best of the best when it comes to getting your explant done right the first time. There are many more options, but when it comes to your health, I only recommend the best. The travel is worth it, if need be.

#4 Customize your Detox and Recovery Healing Protocol Pre- and Post-Explant. Work with an expert who can guide you on properly detoxing the body at the cellular level, physical structure balance, supplements, functional lab work, emotional healing, trauma resolve, confidence, mindset. There is really no *one- size- fits-all* approach to healing, so having it customized to you is paramount.

I highly advise against just taking the same supplements your friend does, that you read about online, those recommended at a health-food store and even caution against taking supplements, bioidenticals, cleanse protocols, etc. from a functional medicine doctor that doesn't specialize in BII, nor has gone through it themselves. BII healing is a unique animal, let's just say we're unicorns. Detox is best alongside a coach, especially to keep you on track, because with explant detox, you will likely want to quit...many times. This will help you dig deeper and having experts on your team who have been in your shoes will help you craft your personal roadmap back to optimal health. I recommend working on number two until you have a surgery date, then you can work on number four with custom functional labs (beyond mainstream medicine and basic blood work) to put a three- or six-month plan in place. This is what we work on in our Support Groups and Transformational Programs, designed to support and meet you where you're at.

#5 Connect with others who will support you emotionally and physically, be there with you along the journey, lift you up, hold space for you, people who won't tear you down. Online Support groups are great, but there's something to be said about having others (family, friends, pets, churches-- whatever resonates with you) to touch, cry and laugh with *in person*. Oxytocin hormones are low with most of us, so personal connection will get those levels rising. Here's a little cheat sheet roadmap for you:

11 Steps to Reverse Breast Implant Illness the Right way

1. Schedule your Explant Surgery
2. 2-3 months Prior, Create Surgery prep Plan
3. Run Advanced Hormone, Gut & Toxicity Panels
4. Prepare Post Explant Protocol with FDN Coach
5. Stop Supplements 2-3 weeks prior to Explant
6. Eat Super Clean & Avoid 7 Inflammatory Foods
7. Clean up & Eliminate Environmental Toxins
8. Go in STRONG to Explant Surgery
9. 4 weeks Post, Start Detox
10. 8 weeks Post, Begin Gut & Hormone Healing Protocol
11. Continue Healing Journey for 1-2 Years

DianeKazer .com - BII & Explant Detox, Self Love & Healing Solutions

Repeat after me: "Simply explanting will not fix all of my problems." I see this belief sabotage women's healing journeys. Often times, this mindset will render them sicker than when they had the implants in. But-- here's the thing. There are women that still don't feel well six months, one year, three years, even five years post explant. Most often, it's because they didn't prepare their bodies for the stress of surgery; nor did they develop a plan to detox implant residue or other toxins, making it difficult to restore the gut, tissues and hormonal systems—all necessary elements for comprehensive, synergistic healing. A physical cure must also involve a spiritual cleanse of our mindset, thereby removing the limiting beliefs that lead us to implant to begin with.

Some say they feel better, sure... But... Most women cannot even imagine their wellness potential until they practice enough self-love on their bodies that they realize their true potential results in feeling three times better than their current situation. Three times... *At least*! It's all about asking yourself, "Am I cool with just feeling okay, with PMS, sleep issues, low sex drive, extra weight, and numbing out with regular consumption of alcohol, caffeine, over-the-counter and prescription drugs*?"* Or "Do I want to *thrive* and feel *alive?"*

✂Remember: the absence of symptoms does not mean the presence of health.

None of this is your fault sister. We've been conditioned to "just numb the symptoms" and escape the pain. It's an outdated system burning down fast because we're waking up! This book is here to help you see the *reality* of what brings you back to life *fast*. Symptoms of BII cause enough suffering as it is.... After the hell you've been through, you deserve to feel your best *and* live your breast life ever, don't you?

Sanity Check

Going to your doctors, trying to convince them you're not crazy, educating them on BII and then requesting them to run labs they aren't aware of... Is going to stress you out even more—consequently prolonging your healing journey.

Let's clear this up. You *will* go nuts if you try this... I see it in our clients all day long. Just the other day, someone contacted me, frantic and desperate because she spent over $50 thousand dollars on twenty-seven doctors who (frustratingly) didn't "get it."

You'll feel like you've talked to every doctor on the planet. You may even burn out, thinking you've tried everything; when in reality, you're relying on people who have no clue what BII is or how to recover from it.

It's like asking your refrigerator to pour you a glass of wine. Although, by the time this book is published, that MAY actually be a 'thing'.

I want you to feel your *best,* not defeated and more confused. If you want to speak with me about the labs you've done, the protocol you've tried and what kind of support may help you break through, I might be able to help, if we have spaces available. If you want to set up a time to talk, you can go to: dianekazer.com/call

Collecting Your Data and Building Your Case

I used to run several labs prior to explant, but as I started to see the same patterns in virtually every woman, I determined the labs I might recommend to each woman prior to explant vary, but I advise them to keep it simple and only run a few to get the big picture on hormone balance, gut health, and mainly detox and metabolic function. Post explant, I recommend waiting to test at least a month after, until the body calms down.

I realize that's a very controversial and disrupting thing to say, but here's the thing: Regardless of how simple or complex, lab results are extremely limiting. Since your trillion some-odd cells are in a constant state of flux, outcomes change daily and can be misleading. They also cost a lot of money and take time to interpret. One could even argue, they are unnecessary, when working with a skilled practitioner. I started looking deeper into my clients' medical history, family history, trauma, toxic exposure and estimated toxic load. I actually took the time to *talk* to them to assess their health based on how they live, think, move, breath and act.

Additional labs and scans to ask your surgeon about include:

- Standard Blood and lab work (this is standard and they will request for you)

- BIA-ALCL, Pathogen Reports-- post explant (be firm about this one)

- Scans (MRI and Ultrasound)

I am frequently asked about mammograms vs thermograms and here are my thoughts:

In our Support Group, one of our members sent me this question: "I am seriously leaning towards explant and had spoken to my husband about my plan of first getting a mammogram then seeing the surgeon that originally placed the implants. Now I am questioning all of that. Is it safe to even get a mammogram?"

I highly recommend you know the risks before you do this. Here are three key points:

1. According to stopcancerfund.org, breast implants can interfere with the detection of breast cancer by obscuring the mammography image of a tumor and potentially delaying the diagnosis of breast cancer.

2. American Cancer Society warns that the X-rays used in mammograms cannot go through silicone or saline implants well enough to show the underlying breast tissue where your radiologist is looking for signs of cancer.

3. Researchers found 66 reports that mentioned problems with mammography for women with breast implants. The majority (62%) of problems reported were for breast implant rupture.

Implants can interfere with the detection of breast cancer in mammograms, as approximately 55% of breast tumors will be hidden in women with implants, not to mention the increased risk of rupture.

"For every woman the harm of mammograms always outweighs the benefit." Today, this is the consensus among most doctors who researched mammography, especially when considering other advancements, both with labs and screenings.

There are less toxic alternatives, such as ultrasound, MRI, and thermograms, which all have different ways of looking into the body for inflammation, infection and implant rupture. Yet, I have found that cross checking them all leads to greater awareness, especially immediately prior to explant.

I've seen a lot of women experience rupture from mammograms, so *particularly* for women with implants, it appears as though the risk outweighs the benefits.

So, what *are* the benefits, if any, to women, implants or not. According to my friend Veronique Desaulniers of Breast Cancer Conqueror, "By the time they see a lump on a mammogram, it has taken five to eight years to develop. And if a woman follows the ten-year protocol of getting a mammogram every year or every six months, she is exposed to as much radiation as a woman who was in Hiroshima during atomic bomb, if she stood only a mile away from the epicenter. She is getting over five rads of radiation if she follows the traditional methods of mammography."

When you consider both the radiation with compression, mammograms cause a lot of problems. Studies have shown that they can *increase* your risk of cancer. A new study twenty-five-year study that came out in Canada found that "mammograms did not decrease breast mortality rate at all. In fact, they were just as effective as a self-exam."

Travel Vans unveil strategic targeted marketing at Nordstrom and other public shopping malls, showing off their shiny, new 3D mamo technology (tomosynthesis, a.k.a. CAT Scans for breasts). Such equipment utilizes even more powerful ionizing radiation-- two or three times higher than the current 2D digital technology. Now, factor in the cumulative destruction caused by inflammation, DNA damage and breast trauma. What these vans also *won't* tell you is that doctors make a *lot* of money on these scans-- they will lose their jobs if they don't remain compliant and push them on their patients.

In the BII space, MRIs and ultrasounds have proven to be far more effective *and* less risky for women with breast implants. SonoCiné ultrasound technology is an adjunct to mammography for women whose mammograms may be inconclusive due to dense breast tissue and/or implants. There is no danger to damaging the implants with the SonoCine ultrasound like there is with a mammogram.

Western medicine is not trained to lead with these before mammograms, so please know this: if you went to your primary care doctor and expected this approach to treatment, you will be sorely disappointed. The future of medicine is to take health into our own hands, partnering with your doctors and health coaches, rather than putting all of our trust in the medical system.   Your most *powerful* weapon to obtain optimal health is to be informed.

Lab Results Worth Your Money

It's important to note, there are lab tests that fail. This is where I see a lot of women spending several thousands, some over ten thousand dollars on either advanced labs or just a lot of unnecessary labs, mostly prescribed by a doctor or coach who uses the same labs on every patient, no matter the symptoms, and is not familiar with BII, or what labs are critical to discover root cause reasons for why a patient is sick. 9 times out of 10, by the time they discover me, they've already spent most of their savings, are on disability or have a hard time stomaching spending any more on labs, because they have been burned.

"Repeat after me: Labs are supplemental, but the cure is you. You are the supplement you have been waiting for." Hence, your money would be better spent on healing solutions that get you better in a few months, rather than spending years spinning your wheels in various 'specialist' doctor's offices. For example, heavy metal testing does not need to cost you tens of thousands of dollars to decipher with countless practitioners. *Yes*, you're filled with metals, we can assume that (if you've had implants). And there is a perfect, ideal formula that can be determined with accurate information.

Blood tests are superficial and don't tell us a lot about your root cause for illness. You're not going to find healing options by doing more tests with your primary care practitioner. You will leave with more drugs though, possibly even a surgery recommendation to remove another organ. No thanks! Not if we can prevent it.

Blood tests for hormone health are short lived and only a tiny snapshot of the *whole* picture

Some of you have spent $3,000 or more to have just *one* test run – such as a silicone toxicity test, which is irrelevant considering there are *far* more important things to collect data on.

I see *every day* how many labs you ladies have run, and it breaks my heart to know how much you've spent on labs that won't help you obtain the appropriate opportunities to heal permanently and holistically, and (finances considered) economically.

Side Note: I was a financial planner for 8 years, through my 20's, and the biggest financial drain I noticed my clients get hit with was 'unexpected medical expenses'. It accounts for over 50% of financial bankruptcies. This is why I'm so conscious about 'saving you money by choosing the most effective fast tracks to optimal healing and getting to the root causes of them so you don't have to waste any more money on band aids that don't work to treat the real problem'.

Let's talk about the lab tests that *are* worth the investment.

Functional lab work can really help you determine where you're starting on the spectrum of toxicity, pathogens (toxic bugs that deplete your energy), hormone imbalances, liver function, neurotransmitters, etc. and help monitor your progress.

The most relevant heavy metals test available to you would be a Urine Toxic Metals test provoked with DMSA. It requires very specific instructions so that you don't make yourself worse in the process. Without DMSA, you won't see much on this test. Metals are stored in your fat and bone in order to protect your body. They

89

don't come out unless provoked with a chelating agent like DMSA. This is why blood tests for toxicity fall short. Blood is a transportation fluid, not a storage fluid so unless you have an acute exposure (like you were exposed to lead paint or you recently ate fish containing mercury), you won't see anything on a blood test. If you really need to see your level of toxicity in black and white, ask a practitioner or reach out to me and we may be able to help, yet I find it unnecessary prior to explant and especially in the earlier stages of detox since (with implants or not), we are all exposed to super high levels today and should all do a deep cleanse, implants or not. And, it's unlikely you will see heavy metals on a lab representative of what's coming out from the brain. It's very difficult to test for this, because it's difficult to pull metals from the brain, however this is something my protocol helps women accomplish. In other words, having results wouldn't be fully accurate nor would it change my protocol recommendations as a start, unless the plan isn't working, and someone is really sick, which is more of an exception.

Mold: Mold is often discussed in the BII world as a problem with breast implants. Know that, as with anything else, this is not always the case. I want to look at the picture as a whole and not treat everyone as if they're the same. We are all exposed to some form of mold and there are dozens of different kinds of mold in the environment, most of which are beneficial rather than harmful. It's whether or not toxic mold is an issue. Working with a Breast Implant Illness Recovery expert will allow you to assess your individual set of symptoms and history, to determine if mold testing is warranted.

We will also cover when to consider these other labs post explant in the future chapters.

- Gut Panel (Inflammation, Infections, Immune Health, Imbalances)
- Food Sensitivities
- Leaky Gut
- Genetics
- Lyme and other Special Considerations

Meanwhile, it couldn't hurt to ask your surgeon to run a Thyroid – Complete Panel (including antibodies and Reverse T3) and EBV (full panel including early antigen) post explant, yet they likely won't have much advice for you since most surgeons are not FDN or holistic health practitioners, and they may not order it for you, because most don't find use in the data.

Finding a Good Doctor

The first and most important step in restoring your health is getting your breast implants properly removed. This means en bloc explant with complete capsulectomy, regardless of the type of implant. This procedure involves removing the implant with the capsule intact, together as one unit, and making sure no pieces of the capsule are left behind in the body.

The capsule contains a matrix of pro-inflammatory cytokines which are capable of promoting an ongoing systemic inflammatory response. A perfect en bloc serves two purposes: avoid unnecessary silicone or microbial contamination of the pocket and the removal of the capsule, which, if not completely removed, will keep on producing inflammatory cytokines and cause chronic inflammation in our bodies. It's also important to note that the capsule also contains silicone and other toxins found in breast implants woven within its matrix.

I can't stress the importance of a complete capsulectomy enough. I've heard many stories of women needing a second surgery to remove capsule tissue that was not removed with explant, in order to completely restore their health. I have also heard stories where surgeons say they will do an en bloc with complete capsulectomy and the patient wakes up from surgery only to discover that the surgeon did not remove the capsule or only partially removed it. I've also consulted with many women who had issues with their implants, and their doctor replaced the implants, but left the festering capsule intact.

Many surgeons believe it's not necessary to remove the capsule. These surgeons do not believe in, nor understand breast implant illness and many are condescending about it, referring to BII as anecdotal. I highly recommend finding a surgeon who not only believes that breast implant illness is real, but also understands it and can describe the en bloc procedure to you. He/she should also provide you with written details of the procedure that is to be performed for you to sign prior to surgery. Be sure to ask for photos and/or video of your en bloc with capsule intact, your implants without the capsule, and your chest cavity to show that all capsule has been removed. Please, do your homework and be sure to choose a surgeon who is experienced and comfortable with en bloc resection.

What Is En Bloc versus Total Capsulectomy?

Total capsulectomy means that all the capsule is removed. "En bloc" is all at once where both are intact – it *is* a total capsulectomy, but the capsule and implant are removed as a single unit (keeping the implant's potential "mess" from escaping).

If there are mold or toxins or infection inside the capsule, when you open it up to remove the implant, whatever is inside will migrate into your chest cavity, which is quite dangerous, being so close to your heart, thyroid, lymph nodes etc. This could result in you becoming very ill. The surgeons that know their stuff avoid this at all costs, hence why it's important you work with a doctor who has experience, education and an emotional connection to truly help and cares.

Think of your implant as a raw egg inside of a shell. You want to have the entire unbroken egg removed, so that the raw egg doesn't spill out inside of you. You want it all contained. If your surgeon opened the capsule, and it's ruptured, all of the toxins will spill and travel all throughout your body! That's why I shared two pictures of my implants, so you can see the capsule intact (looks like a hamburger) and the implant exposed after he cut the capsule to expose the quality of the implant, ruptured, punctured or intact. Just because it's intact doesn't mean it didn't slowly gel bleed throughout your body. Remember the study where 21 percent of women experienced gel bleed of silicone from their capsule, without their knowledge and without symptoms to report?

The capsule, which is scar tissue your body creates around the implant to protect you, is what adheres to the rib cage. Anytime your implants are under the muscle, you can count on the capsule sticking to rib cage, which is exactly what happened to me, and is why my ribs were constantly out of place and why no chiropractic adjustment, massage, physical therapy, nor acupuncture could ever fix my pain.

Should your silicone implant be disintegrated, or your saline implant have mold in it, you want to be sure the capsule remains intact surrounding it so that you don't potentially expose your body to toxins/mold.

Just as important is total capsulectomy because you want all that capsule, scar tissue and silicone removed. Trust that the surgeon you choose will make the smallest incision they can, while safely removing the implant and capsule.

If you have any capsule left due to being worried about a scar you will remain sick or get sicker.

Booby buyer beware: From a woman in my group "My plastic surgeon just said he would replace my implants and while in there he would just clean up the capsule. He said I would not like being without implants because I would be totally flat. Has anybody had this problem?" (Palm to forehead.)

Another eye roll: "The patient coordinator really made it seem like a total capsulectomy was fine and that an en bloc was such a big deal and was a waste of spending the extra money."

So, friends… know what you're up against when you start this journey. Learn to be very firm with your wants, clear with your needs and have a team who really gets it to support you along the way. Many of my clients called me crying, frustrated and I told them to hand the phone over to the technician or whomever they were talking to. Within seconds, we had it cleared up. People aren't trying to be d*cks, they're just usually misinformed, so be mindful about who you vent at and use compassion, rather than trying to teach them everything about what you are going through. Your hormones will thank you!

Which surgery should I do? Explant only? Lift? Fat transfer?

I have already talked a lot about explant and en bloc, which is a given for your surgery if you have BII and wish to recover.

As far as further options, you have choice. You can a la carte to your surgery, a lift and/or fat transfer. Let me explain further.

Breast Lift - I have been interviewed hundreds of times on BII and it can get serious, heavy and gory describing the symptoms and journey, as you can imagine. When I am asked about the surgery I decided upon and how I went about choosing, I tell them this. My implants were so big, weighing in at 1.2 pounds each that I had 'downward facing nipples'. I couldn't see them anymore, so I opted for a lift. In general, most surgeons will suggest a lift if you had larger implants for a longer period of time, but it's ultimately your choice.

Fat Transfer - I also opted for a fat transfer because I was afraid that if I just explanted and got a lift, I would revert back to my pre-implant breasts were quite small and deflated. Once I learned how to properly fitness train for performance with weights, cross training and optimum strength training, I burned fat fast, and I know I will always keep that off, because I challenge my body. Therefore, I opted for fat transfer to volumize my breasts. It was an extra $5,000 or so, but for reasons stated above and I also wanted to endure the experience, so I could write about it in my book and help you, I decided to do it all at once.

I was told the surgery would take 8 hours.

Gulp! 8 HOURS?

That's a long time to be under anesthesia.

But I was reassured I was in good hands and since I had worked on optimizing my body, endocrine system, lymphatic drainage and detox systems, I felt like I would be ok.

Fat transfer is where your surgeon performs liposuction on areas where your body stores fat such as your thighs, buttocks, back, belly and arms.

At 19% body fat, I didn't have much fat to spare, but was told it wasn't a problem.

My main question was: just how much volume would we be able to 'harvest' from my fat pockets to volumize my breasts?

These were my results, 4 weeks after my surgery:

- Fat Transfer 100CC's to each breast
- Lost 4% body fat (19% to 15%)
- Lost 8 pounds (from 149 to 141)
- Went from a DD to a Small C, 500CC breasts, weighing 1.2 pounds each GONE

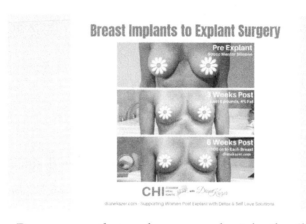

Breast Implants to Explant Surgery

Pre Explant
500cc Mentor Silicone

3 Weeks Post
Lost 6 pounds, 4% Fat

6 Weeks Post
100 cc to Each Breast
dianekazer.com

CHI CLEANSE HEAL IGNITE ™ with *Diane Kazer*

dianekazer.com · Supporting Women Post Explant with Detox & Self Love Solutions

Do you see that rash on my chest in the 'before' picture? Yeah, those don't happen anymore. Neither do many other symptoms on my pre-explant list...which I am finding the list is getting smaller as I progress along the Detox Phases I teach in my BII Healing & Recovery Program – Cleanse, Heal, Ignite.

4 weeks after those statistics, and I lost another 6 pounds. I was 8 weeks post explant, and lost 15 pounds total, lighter than I was in high school. I was thrilled!

And you know...I was also very proud. I celebrated my courage, recovery and freedom! The day I weighed in at 135 was the day after I climbed to the top of Mt Baldy, a goal of mine for a while. It was July 28, 8 weeks after my surgery.

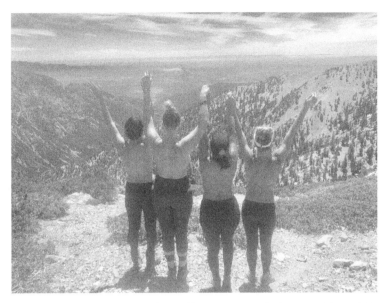

By that time, I was literally on top of the world, spiritually, emotionally, physically. Not financially so much, because I had just spent $15,000 on my surgeries and medical bills but hey, what's your health and silicone freedom worth right?

I had also celebrated by taking a scuba diving in Cabo, riding my horse again, and began playing soccer. As you'll soon read, August 16th, 10 weeks after my explant is when everything changed for me.

Recovery time

Keep in mind that if you opt to do fat transfer, it is one of the most painful experiences you'll probably ever endure and is also why I wouldn't recommend it again. I'm not super convinced on fat transfer as a great idea for women, especially who are already suffering with illness, because first of all, I was injured ten weeks after mine, and second, I developed some pretty significant fat necrosis, which is dead fat tissue, where the body essentially stops sending blood flow to the fat placed into your breast pockets. Chances are higher if you wear tight fitting compression garments, which I did, and we are advised to post surgery. Fat necrosis is not usually a health concern or issue for cancer, but it is slightly painful and uncomfortable, and can also deform your breasts. Mine weren't but I was definitely concerned about it.

Upon doing an ultrasound, we discovered I had it in both breasts so my dear friend, Dr Juan Garcia, performed PRP (Platelet Rich Plasma) on me. It wasn't my intention for this trip, but I had gone to Tijuana, Mexico to get IV C, glutathione and biological dentistry treatments. It turned out I was in for a treat, as that weekend, I developed an entire explant, pre and post healing protocol with the head doctor at their clinic because within two weeks after my PRP injections, the lumps were gone.

My final recommendation to women is this. Do Surgery #1 where you just explant, and if you desire, a lift. See how you feel, let your body heal and if you don't like the appearance of how your breasts settled in, go in for Surgery #2 six to twelve months later and get a fat transfer. Warning to the warrior from the wise: Be very cautious as some surgeons are very aggressive with their fat transfers, to the point that they are able to create a D cup from an A cup. I do not believe it is safe, nor advisable, especially since the weight distribution for a woman's body was not created for that much extra weight on the front, so it's going back to the original problem the woman had when she had her implants, which could negatively impact the curve of her back.

Fat Transfer Considerations for Mastectomy Patients

If you have had your breast/s removed completely and implants replaced them, keep in mind fat transfer is an option, but as of now, it involves about 5 procedures to gain the desired effect. It's still a new and emerging procedure, and as time goes on, advancements are being developed to simplify this process and offer less toxic alternatives, like prosthetics, stem cells to rebuild breasts, PRP and more. For now, grafting is the gold standard. And because fat grafting is so new, no large clinical studies have been done on the procedure, and the ones that have been done involve fewer than 100 women and the average follow-up time is less than 4 years.

In many cases, the fat injected into the breasts gets reabsorbed by the body over time, so they may lose some volume. This is why some plastic surgeons initially may add more fat than you think you need. For example, I lost about 50% of mine, about 50 CC's of the 100 CC's placed into each breast.

If fat grafting doesn't work and you decide you want a flap reconstruction, you may have already used up an important source of tissue such as the belly area. These are all things to keep in mind, so be sure to consult with a specialized doctor in Flap procedures, who are familiar with the many reconstruction options, and decide together.

After one type of fat grafting procedure, an external tissue expander called a Brava device is worn for several weeks before and after the fat grafting. The Brava device is like a bra with plastic cones for cups, which put suction on the breast area to expand the tissue and create a matrix for the fat to live and mold into, with the idea being to maintain the breast tissue volume added. In one study, women who didn't wear the Brava device as directed had their breast volume decrease nearly twice as much as women who wore the Brava device.

Depending on your reconstructed goal breast size, you may have to undergo multiple fat grafting procedures done over a period of months, usually under general anesthesia.

According to BreastCancer.org:

The advantages of fat grafting are:

- It uses your own tissue instead of an implant.
- Fat is removed from an area where you don't want it.
- Many women report that their fat-graft-reconstructed breast has some sensation and feels soft, much like the other unreconstructed breast.

The disadvantages of fat grafting are:

- No large clinical studies with long-term follow-up have been done on fat grafting; while small studies report good results, we don't know if this technique will work for all women and we also don't know how long the results will last.

- Depending on which surgeon you choose to do the procedure, you may be required to wear the Brava device or another type of external tissue expander for 4 or more weeks before the fat injections and for several weeks after.

- It may require 4 to 6 individual sessions to get the best potential results.

- The injected fat may be reabsorbed by the body and you may lose some or all of the breast volume over time.

- Because some fat cells can stimulate cell growth, some doctors are concerned that fat injected into the breast area may cause dormant breast cancer cells to grow; research needs to be done to find out if this is true.

- Some of the fat injected into the breast area may die, which is called "necrosis." Symptoms of necrosis may include pain and bleeding, the skin turning dark blue or black, numbness, fever, and sores that ooze a bad-smelling discharge or pus.

- You may exhaust a key tissue source for a future flap reconstruction if fat grafting doesn't work.

This is a plan you should work with your doctor to hash out. Don't forget to bring with you the list of questions to ask your surgeon, take the Neurotoxic quiz on my website and if you decide to explant and rebuild your breasts, prepare wisely for it using the recommendations in this book. If it were me, I wouldn't want to take the risk having implants in my body, knowing what I know now, and I would aim for reconstruction, but that is ultimately your choice.

Is it just my implants causing all my symptoms?

NO! It's Not JUST your Breast Implants making you Sick. It's also...

1. Improperly Filtered Water
2. Poor diet, deplete in micronutrients & balanced macros
3. Toxic Personal Care products
4. Shame based thoughts & ensuing emotions
5. Poor air quality
6. ElectroSmog and Wifi Radiation
7. Too much or too little exercise
8. Disconnection from Nature
9. Insufficient sunlight & Vitamin D
10. Toxic Relationships, Friendships, Partnerships

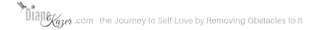
DianeKazer.com - the Journey to Self Love by Removing Obstacles to It

"Can you really blame the implants exclusively?" Was one of the many questions that popped into my inbox after I shared my article on my Social Media channels: "33 Reasons *Not* to Get Breast Implants Your Doctor Didn't Warn You About."

My response to her: *Great* question!

Of course, implants play a *huge* role in our health issues and cognitive decline. They're a permanent drip of toxicity threatening our immune system at high alert twenty-four/seven trying to do whatever they can do to attack them and detox them out of our bodies. This by its true definition is *auto immune disease*. Self-attack on a foreign object from the outside the body comes into contact with on the inside.

Our body doesn't hate us, it *loves* us and is literally trying to save our lives. God doesn't make junk nor do our systems respond by accident with the language of symptoms. This is the compassionate journey we must walk back toward our hearts on the path of explant and beyond.

Breast implants (both silicone and saline) wear down the immune system, deplete our hormones, drain our brain, and destroy our gut! Total body shut-down!

But, that's just part of the puzzle.

You can't just remove the implants without properly detoxing your body, repairing all of the organs it disabled, and reprogramming the mind that said we weren't beautiful enough before we implanted.

We must consider *all* potential areas of toxicity and trauma today.

Apart from implants, here are the main ones. Removing implants will resolve some symptoms, but the others are supported by detox, then rebuilding and restoring the body, mindset and emotional trauma with a customized approach considering these factors! "Most women don't get better with explant alone."

Addressing *all* of these key areas is what this book and the work I do to support women in their transformation are all about. It is what gets women *finally* across the finish line after years of trying either one thing at a time or multiple things inconsistently that don't complement one another.

It's not just about removing the implants. Having implants in our body causes a *lot* of long-term damage to tissues, organs, and our psychology. I wish it were as easy as removing them and everything gets better, but it just doesn't. For most women 60-70 percent of symptoms will resolve, but not all. Then, what about the other 20-30 percent nagging symptoms? There are two things happening here: Post explant, we all need to detox, rebuild and heal from implant residue and/or clean up other areas of her life. Usually I find it's a combination of *both*.

And depending on the woman, her genes, how long she has had her implants, the symptoms may take a while to cease. The genetic weaknesses such as MTHFR, HLA-B27, HLA-DR52, and HLA-DR53 gene mutations, deserve some special attention.

The question to ask yourself is:

"Am I ok with waiting for months, years hoping symptoms may go away *or* would I rather rebuild my body ASAP, so I don't risk possible long-term damage *and* work on detoxing the things I know all women with breast implants suffer from which is heavy-metal, gut bugs, poor confidence and hormonal chaos?"

Remember: Breast implants are toxic to our bodies, but there is a *lot* else to consider that most aren't today, implants or not.

You know how I said I lost fifteen pounds in eight weeks? It wasn't just because I explanted. It was all of the work I did to prepare before and to detox and heal after, the most important being:

1. Boosting metabolism and optimizing minerals

2. Balancing blood sugar with healthy food and a stable mood

3. Opening up detox pathways

4. Optimizing digestion

5. Nourishing the tissues and organs

In that order.

There is a handful of women who are getting this dialed in right and are getting better fast. You just have to ask yourself how important it is to you. This list may look overwhelming to you, but when you have a solid team to simplify this for you and aim to address all of these things, at once customized to you and only you and not a template protocol, your body will rejoice and heal quickly.

BEYOND REMOVING BREAST IMPLANTS, THIS MUST ALL BE ADDRESSED TO RESTORE HEALTH

HEAVY METAL DETOX
SILICONE & SALINE DETOX
GLYPHOSATE DETOX
OTHER CHEMICALS DETOX
XENOESTROGEN DETOX (PLASTIC, PARABENS, PESTICDES)
LEAKY GUT HEALING
INFECTION REMOVAL (CANDIDA, PARASITES, BACTERIA, VIRAL)
IMMUNE SYSTEM STRENGTHENING
BODY TISSUE RESTORATION
RE-MINERALIZATION
REBUILDING NUTRIENT DEFICIENCIES
INFLAMMATION REDUCTION DEEPER IN THE BODY
CELLULAR OPTIMIZATION
METABOLISM MODULATION
CHILDHOOD TRAUMA RESOLVE
INSECURITY & POOR CONFIDENCE
BELIEF SYSTEMS
HEALTHY BOUNDARIES
LIFESTYLE
SELF CARE
SELF WORTH
SELF LOVE AND CELL HEALTH!

CHI CLEANSE HEAL HOUSE *with DivaKaye* .com

Getting Insurance to Work with You

I paid $128 for my explant. This is about cultivating courage to speak up for what you deserve, like a boss and then celebrating your explant co-pay. I busted my bum to earn this one. And it was SO worth it.

My final breakdown was this: my surgeon, Dr. Strawn was paid $570 for the explant portion of the surgery by Blue Shield, and my portion was $128.00 (approximately 20 percent). It's all about knowing how to research the doctors listed on your in-network surgeons, then starting a case with a doctor you trust that will go to bat with and for you.

Here are some things to rely on during this process:

108

- Keep being loud.

- Do not take no for an answer.

- Be a f*cking warrior, woman.

- Stand up for what you believe is right.

For *this* is what happens when you *do*.

When I first started my explant journey, my insurance company was exhausting and clueless to work with. Every time I called, I got a different answer. I wanted to bang my head against the wall. For real.

Then I had to go through all the hoops: ultrasound, MRI, doctors' appointments, blood work, etc. I filed a claim through an explant insurance-approved doctor (Dr Strawn in Newport Beach, CA).

And still they denied me.

To which I replied "Oh, hell no!"

I persisted and got my doctor's staff to work with me by sending a rebuttal letter stating the reasons why I thought my explant should be covered:

I'd been taking pain meds to no relief, had multiple and repeated rashes unresolved with prednisone, was doing physical therapy, had capsular contracture (this one weighs in the most for approval if you can get your doctor to prove you have it, especially grade four), etcetera, etcetera.

That letter got me a peer-to-peer insurance-doctor-to-surgeon session so my surgeon could go to battle with me to get my insurance approved, which he did.

Not because he's the best doctor ever, though I do believe he is amazing. But because I *fought for myself and didn't take 'No' for answer.*

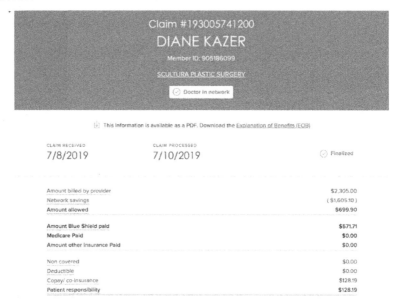

I worked with the best in the industry to learn everything I could about Breast Implant Illness, what it is, how to have my best shot at getting it covered by insurance, how to find the best doctor, how to best prepare my body for surgery, how to detox after surgery and how to prepare my mind and heart for the changes ahead, with my main goal being:

- How to pass the buck,
- Lead this mission and

- Help *you* ladies so you don't have to do all this work yourself.

Because it's freaking hard and confusing and with as sick as so many of us are in this process, my goal was to walk through this fire of overwhelming details, because I know I was created for this stuff ... so I could lead you all through the fire holding buckets of water.

Celebrate that this is possible for all of us, when you have the right leadership.

There are two ways to do it: the hard way and the easy way. If you want the hard way, have at it. But, if you want the easy way, I've cracked the code and what joy it is to watch the ladies I'm working with fly through it, so they can enjoy life instead of figuring it all out themselves.

If you are looking to shortcut this crazy maze, I am here to help. I created this BII explant to empowerment and recovery blueprint so all you have to do is follow the plan customized exactly to you. I will stand with you, even when you're feeling weak and you can't fight anymore.

Other women in I've worked with have shared similar stories of bypassing insurance, making it 'easier' on themselves and paying out of pocket to save the hassle:

"I did not feel confident with the in-network doctors, so I paid for mine myself. My husband was supportive and said to get a good surgeon and not one that didn't even believe in *capsules*. I would have loved to fight and get it covered but in the end my health was degrading. The rest was covered by credit card. My explant surgeon was worth every penny. I am so happy that there are positive insurance stories out there. You get'em, ladies! One day hopefully explants will be covered."

But here's the thing. If you knew what to do to get your procedure covered by insurance, saving you around $5,000, wouldn't you like to use that savings toward bringing yourself and your health back to life quickly with a cleanse, heal, ignite protocol?

I'm not an expert at insurance, but I am passionate about fighting for what I believe is *right* and I am an expert at getting you ready for surgery and helping you recover afterward.

Keep fighting, ladies. Your voice matters! And you deserve to be covered for this procedure. They didn't give AF about you, nor your health by properly researching the long-term safety of implants, so this financial burden should lie on them.

Chapter 5: Preparing for Exorcism, I Mean Explant

Myth: The body detoxes heavy metals, silicone and saline all by itself. I don't need to do anything other than remove my breast implants because it will take care of itself in time. Time heals all things.

Truth: It takes one or two years of concerted effort of an individualized protocol to detox properly from toxin leakage caused by implants, then heal damaged gut tissues and hormone glands.

There is a huge misconception in the BII space and myth of 'Overnight healing' which is not what it seems and sets a lot of women up for failure, having expectations that this will and should be them. Take a look at my before and after photo one week apart. Sure, my inflammation dropped, life came back into my eyes and my skin improved, but this was after heavy doses of antibiotics, pain medications and anesthesia. The reality is, for most women, they tend to feel better for a few weeks or a few months, then symptoms return, some new, some old. Overall, most feel 'better' but a huge part of this process, as is with anything, to manage your expectations, since disappointment can and usually creates more suffering than toxins themselves.

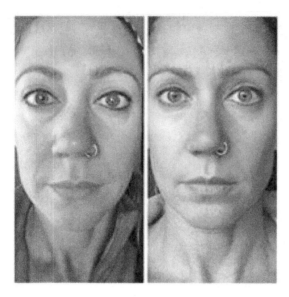

My 7 days before and morning after explant mug shot

Let's talk about how you can heal fast by preparing for a healthy, successful explant with the best chance of fast recovery optimizing diet, rest, movement, mindset, and reducing stress.

For sake of simplicity, because this is not a diet or recipe book, I am going to keep this as straightforward as possible. Eating healthy will be critical to prepare your body to be strong for explant and to expedite your healing post explant because there's not a whole lot you can do prior to explant in the way of Advanced Detox, with the root-cause toxic offender still in your body. You don't want to do that because you run the risk of simply stirring up toxins more. Doing things like sitting in hot saunas could increase the risk of gel bleed of your implants. This is unique to each individual and depends on the type of sauna used as well, so it's not a blaket statement to say 'all women with breast implants should avoid saunas' as it depends on a lot of things.

What *is* safe to do in the way of detox prior to explant is still developing in the research and not 100 percent clear, but to be safe, the best place to start is to support your body with healthy foods that your body agrees with, so let's start there!

Top Ten Pre-Explant Foundational Guidelines

1. Mindset is key – explore your soul goal (coming in the next chapters), intentions, prayers, I-am statement, and self-love promises to avoid self-betrayal. Remove "perfect," "fail", and "overwhelm" from your vocabulary.

2. Self-love – take breaks. Know your limits. Communicate your needs. I teach clients Self Love Sunday so it's a given every week and develops consistency. Knowing there's an upcoming 'break' in the busy-ness of life is so important. Live it in gratitude, a Full Spectrum sauna, nature, essential oils, massage, love making ... whatever gets your heart behind the wheel. When I work 1 on 1 with clients, we focus on this a great deal because what I have found most in the BII space, is a lot of women who have never learned to love themselves as we are and put ourselves last in the self-care category. In fact, a recent study revealed women put themselves dead last on the priority list. Are you ready to end that culturally indoctrinated habit?

3. Boundaries – Practice self-respect by protecting your body, schedule, and heart like a warrior. Protect your cleanse, heal, ignite process like a bad ass. You can express and implement commitments you have to yourself and achieve that balance with commitments to others, without being a bitch, you feel me? Passive aggressive communication usually stems from a childhood where you felt unheard, so it comes out a bit bitchy, especially when the other person isn't respecting your needs. Anyone who doesn't respect your compassionate, clearly communicated boundaries is not a friend. You may have heard "Those who do not honor your boundaries, lack boundaries themselves". This is a huge part of the emotional rehab I have supported clients toward freedom, and it's connected to the reason most of us got implants to begin with.

4. Sleep seven to nine hours per night, without interruptions, ideally from 10 p.m. to 6 a.m. If you have 'sleep issues' there could be a lot going on, and I'll lay out solutions in later chapters. You CAN have quality sleep without needing to sedate yourself with toxic sleep medications, that in my experience working with BII women, worsen symptoms, because of the damage it causes the body and brain.

5. Drink three to four liters of clean, filtered water daily. Avoid ice and drinking more than four ounces during a meal. Ice causes the pores of the digestive track to shrink, thereby reducing absorption of quality nutrients from food. Add lemon for extra liver love.

6. Get moving. But not too much. Three to four times per week for thirty minutes at a time is ideal. Avoid steady state cardio and shoot for HIIT and body or weight bearing exercises. Also important is to have your Hormones properly tested to explore the state of your Endocrine system. Many women with BII are very sick, and high intensity exercise aggravate that through cortisol bursts, negatively impacting sex and sleep hormones and shunting cortisol away from reducing inflammation as a result of breast implants. I highly recommend going deeper to have this all customized, beyond blood testing, especially for hormones because it lacks the big picture of what hormones are actually getting used by the body vs just produced. I'll talk more about specific testing I recommend in future chapters. They're Game Changers.

7. Chill out when you eat – be present with your meals and avoid doing multiple things at once. Your body won't be able to digest optimally if you give it too many jobs. Digestion uses up about 70% of our caloric intake every day, so it's critical we make this easy, so your body has more energy for other things like detox and healing. Masticate my love! That means chew! Twenty-five chews for the high fiber, protein dense foods. And for protein shakes or drinks, hold your first sip in your mouth for twenty-five seconds. Swish it around, hold it on and under your tongue, which triggers your digestive glands to start releasing acid, bile and enzymes.

8. Avoid grazing, we're not gazelles, LOL. Try to eat every three to four hours if possible. If your meals don't last that long, add

more fat and fiber to your next meal. Everyone's fat and fiber needs are different, and it really depends on your genetics, gut microbes, activity demands, toxicity levels, age where you're at along your BII journey and more. A way to go deeper to customize this is to explore your gut health through a Stool test. I see the majority of clients working with doctors who get this wrong, and it bums me out because I know how hard you work to find answers. Not to worry, I'll get to that in future chapters.

9. Journal your progress, so you can learn to listen to and observe patterns for what your body is trying to say, what it likes, dislikes and are not yet sure of. Track your stool, period, urine cycles, hunger, digestion responses, how you feel when you rise, go to sleep, before and after work outs, etc. Ideally, you're working with a practitioner who can help you make sense of your symptoms. I've created some great tools to accomplish this in my online programs that have helped thousands of women learn more about their body and to develop a connection with her intuition, by learning the language of her symptoms. It's one of the greatest gifts you can give yourself.

10. JERF – just eat real food. Avoid: processed foods (think things in boxes). 70% of foods at the grocery store are just that…and are a huge source of stress for most of us today!

I have several programs and recipe books if you need guidelines on what's healthy, tasty and convenient. And ways to go deeper to customize that if you need guidance or are like me and prefer to have it all customized to save me time, money and energy on things that aren't for me or even make things worse.

Because it can be hard today with convenient, fast, on the go food everywhere. The idea is to real, fresh, local food. Food without labels. If anything, less than five ingredients. Stay conscious to work toward avoiding artificial anything.

No "concentrate" juice – eat whole fruits instead (you need the fiber). Avoid GMO's. Prioritize organic, grass-fed meat, wild-caught, sustainably raised fish.

"If you don't know what it is or how to pronounce it, it's probably going to take more life force from you to break it down than provide energy and vitality to you."

You can look at this one of two ways:

• Wow this is really restrictive. I can't eat much of anything anymore.

• Wow this is really simple. Buy Organic. Go to Farmer Markets. Shop the perimeter.

Avoid stuff in the middle. Eat like we did 100 years ago. Eat like a human is supposed to. Things our body recognizes. Nothing it doesn't. "If you don't recognize it, your body won't recognize it either" And things our body doesn't recognize turns into sickness and symptoms; disease and death. The more alive food you eat, the more alive you'll feel and the faster you'll heal on the other side of explant.

I practice an 80/20 rule. 80 percent of my food, meals and snacks are comprised of real food, and 20 percent I allow to be snacks, but it's so easy now to honor that with clean food. There's a myriad of potato chips, chocolate, wine, coffee organic options so when I indulge, I opt for the healthiest version that my inner child snacker is craving. However, I do avoid gluten and soy like the plague, and I recommend you do too. Allow me to explain.

Eat Clean and Limit These Six Inflammatory Foods

1. Sugar – stick to no more than 50g per day. 5g per 100 cal
2. Artificial sweeteners, colors, ingredients
3. Gluten and inflammatory grains ... instead I recommend eating seeds and nuts, quinoa, hemp, chia, buckwheat, etc.
4. Soy – it's very estrogenic, which women with BII usually already have high levels of estrogen because the implants are xenoestrogens.
5. GMO's - especially corn which is loaded with glyphosate and mold that adds to most women's already existing levels of high mold caused by the implants
6. PUFA's found in industrial oils such as canola oil, vegetable oil, corn oil, peanut oil, soy oil, etc. These are extremely inflammatory and clog our eliminatory pathways.

Corn is mostly GMO today and can be found in most products on the market in the form of citric acid, powdered sugar, corn flour, tea bags, paper plates, disposable cutlery, fructose, corn meal, corn oil, corn syrup, dextrin and dextrose, fructose, lactic acid, malt, mono- and diglycerides, monosodium glutamate, shredded cheese, seasonings, supplements, sorbitol, and starch, as well as many others. Obviously, it's impossible to avoid, so I recommend you don't obsess over it, like a crazy perfectionist and just do your best to educate yourself.

Also limit:

• Eating out. There are few restaurants today that offer the diet recommendations I'm providing you here. If you *must* eat out, take a binder like activated charcoal/clay blends, and at best, go gluten- and soy-free, plus lay low on the sugar and alcohol.

• Commercially raised animals and opt for organic, grass-fed, happy animals without hormones. I eat maybe one meat meal per day.

• Caffeine – a Super popular swap recipe for this that thousands of women love more than their morning coffee is a recipe I made to curb my own addiction called the Metabolic Mocha. You'll find the recipe and videos for how to make it on my Resources section.

• Alcohol (except negligible amounts in Kombucha). Maybe one glass of Organic red wine per week to maintain your sanity but anything else will be added burden on the liver.

Here are some healthy swaps:

Baby step your way up to familiarizing yourself with these healthier versions of the most common fake foods I refer to as "pheud" in the SAD (Standard American Diet). The sooner you and your family are off this junk, the better everything will be.

- Instead of: soy sauce

Try: organic tamari (still soy, but wheat free and fermented) or coconut aminos (preferred choice)

- Instead of: dairy milk or soy milk

Try: homemade nut milk recipe or store-bought refrigerated nut milk

- Instead of: white bread or any gluten containing bread

Try: coconut wraps, seaweed strips, lettuce wraps using collards, bib lettuce, or kale

- Instead of: white cane sugar

Try: raw honey, monk fruit, 100 percent maple syrup, organic stevia

- Instead of: processed oils like canola oil

Try: coconut oil, avocado oil or olive oil

- Instead of: milk chocolate

Try: raw dark cocoa products

- Instead: dairy ice cream or yogurt

Try: coconut store bought or homemade "ice cream" made with frozen banana, nut milk, and maple syrup/stevia

- Instead of: white rice, couscous, white pasta

Try: quinoa, quinoa *pasta*, buckwheat, amaranth, zoodles (zucchini noodles), spaghetti squash

- Instead of: regular butter

Try: grass-fed butter or good quality ghee (traditional, clarified butter)

It can be overwhelming to read all of this and implement it, which is why I created my online program 'The Warrior Cleanse' to teach you how to make it routine, habit, affordable, realistic and fun!

More Advanced Diet Tips

Nutrient Dense Food

If there's one thing I despise about the health, yoga, fitness and life coach field, it's dogmatic, exclusionary, template advice that is prescribed to work for everyone. Although there are foods that I recommend everyone avoid, there will never be one diet that works for you all the time. Many things will change and go in cycles, such as your period, the seasons, where you live/travel, your activity levels, detox needs, you get the idea? Many of my BII clients have done well trying the Auto Immune Paleo Diet, Anti Inflammatory Diet (which are essentially the foods I've recommended to you), the Low Histamine Diet, Keto or combination of some of them. It's essentially what I recommend in the Warrior Cleanse, and take it a step further when I see their labs to customize foods, macros, feeding cycles, etc. I have seen vegan diet work okay for some, yet most I see eating this way are high-carb loaded, eating lots of gluten and soy, which are extremely inflammatory and don't offer much in the way of amino acids to help heal tissues that are compromised in us with BII.

Quality Water

You may have heard it before: drink half of your body weight in ounces per day of filtered water every day. This will keep your detox pathways working more efficiently by assisting the kidneys in filtering the blood when your detox program increases the amount of toxins removed from places like your lymphatic system. Make sure you are not drinking tap or bottled water as they both increase the overall burden on the body. Bottled water contains endocrine disrupting chemicals like BPA. Don't let those labels "BPA free" fool you; there are many other forms of bisphenol used in the making of plastics and cans, like BPS. Tap water is filled with toxins that will add to your toxic load. My recommendation is to use a whole house water filtration system, which you can learn more about in the resources section on my website. Products are always evolving, so I have created a section on my website, where I update my recommendations, so you are always abreast of the best of the best for you and your family.

The Original Mineral Water - Sole

In order to detoxify, your body needs energy and to produce energy, your body needs minerals. Minerals nourish your adrenals and thyroid, your main organs of energy production. Did you know 98% of your hormones are made from minerals? We deplete our mineral levels due to internal and external stress, including toxic exposures like those found in breast implants. I love to drink sole water for restoring minerals especially before and after infrared saunas. All you do is simply fill ¼ of a large mason jar with Himalayan Sea Salt and fill it to the top with filtered water. Let it sit overnight, shake it up and then add 1 tsp of the Sole to an 8 oz glass of water every morning on an empty stomach. I suggest mineral rebalancing and addressing your specific mineral deficiencies due to heavy metal toxicity after explant, but for now this will suffice. If you would like to explore mineral levels, mineral ratios and heavy metal toxicity levels in your body, ask a holistic health practitioner, or you can reach out to me and my online clinic to discuss.

Eliminate Environmental Stressors

It may surprise you to know that your indoor air is up to 100 times more polluted than outdoor air. This is because of high levels of environmental stressors, common toxins found in your home, work, and outside environment that have negative health impacts. Things like household cleaning products, antiperspirants, air fresheners, scented candles, perfumes, makeup, hair care, electronics, furniture, carpets, etc. can all be a source of toxic exposure. Gradually swapping these conventional products for healthier non-toxic alternatives helps decrease the toxic burden on the body. The best resource for cleaning up your home environment with healthier products is Environmental Working Group: www.ewg.org Also consider swapping your Beauty and Personal Care products with non-toxic or lower toxic sources which I elaborate on deeply in my online programs you'll see in the resources section.

Beauty, I Mean Booby Sleep

Quality sleep is incredibly important for proper detoxification and healing. While you're sleeping is when your body is actually doing the detoxification work, did you know that? Getting at least eight hours of quality sleep is recommended any time, but especially when preparing to undergo the stress of surgery and post recovery. You can find more details on Sleep Hacks in future chapters.

Preparing for Post-Explant Detoxing

Gall Bladder and Liver Love

Once you have taken these steps to prepare your body, you can begin the deeper work in preparation for detoxing after explant in the following order. A large portion of the toxins processed by the liver are excreted into the bile which is also made in the liver. The bile is concentrated in the gallbladder and eventually makes its way through the intestines to be eliminated in the stool. It is essential to have the bowels moving frequently before you start any detox program, or the toxins can be reabsorbed into the body if the transit time through the bowel is slow. This is one of the number One Fails I've seen in my ten years leading detox programs, is they force their body to begin releasing toxins before they have a literal exit strategy, which has the opposite effect they intended.

My golden rule for guiding my clients through a detox program is they should have 2-3 'banana poo' bowel movements a day. While that may seem like a lot to someone who only goes once every few days, it's actually quite healthy and I don't have to tell you that having a good release, is truly 'the shit', especially when you feel a sense of emotional freedom at the same time and you've truly 'let that shit go'. Remember, what's "normal for you" or what your Western doctor told you is 'normal', may not actually be normal or healthy for optimal health.

Here's why: Whenever you're lagging on poop, you're not only constipated with unhealthy dead bacteria and other pathogens, you're also constipated with the toxins your liver has worked so hard to release. After **bile** enters and passes down the small intestine, about **90% of bile** salts are reabsorbed into the bloodstream through the wall of the lower small intestine. The liver extracts these **bile** salts from the blood and re-secretes them back into the **bile**. **Bile** salts go through this cycle about 10 to 12 times a day.

So, what this means is, you're not detoxing, you're simply 'moving toxins from one safe place to a less safe place in the body.

What you're not excreting, you're reabsorbing, which is bad news because once toxins are released from the areas they are stored in a 'low danger zone' (such as fat cells), they are now running free without being attached to a transport binding molecule, with the potential to cause more harm, akin to prisoners getting out of jail prematurely. These toxic prisoners are now free to roam their way into 'high danger zones' around your body, vital for survival, such as the brain, organs and heart. The brain is the highest danger zone, comprised of 60 percent fat, the preferred storage site of toxins, especially heavy metals, which cross the blood brain barrier, especially with women who have BII due to increased inflammation and infection, medication use as well as physical injury.

Brain fog is super common with anyone who is neurotoxic, not to mention mental diseases relative to toxins in the brain such as the Alzheimer's and dementia aluminum connection as well as the Anxiety and Panic attack Mercury connection. This is why women with BII feel like we're literally losing our mind, because our brain is neurotoxic, backlogged with toxins and metals from our breast implant gel bleed and beyond. I recommend taking the Neurotoxic Quiz found in the Resources section to check your score and map out your Detox and healing journey to Cleanse, Heal and Ignite your way to your new, upgraded self both before and after explant, which will look different to minimize Herx'ing. A 'Herxeimer' reaction is where your body detoxes faster than your body is able to release toxins, and your body experiences less than pleasant symptoms that make you want to quit.

This is another Cleanse Fail I see all the time, and why I recommend you work with a skilled practitioner both before and after explant. I learned this one the hard way, which is why I wrote this book and work with clients one on one to help you avoid the pain I endured. The more toxic you are and the more imbalanced your hormones are, the greater damage your metabolism has experienced. From my clinical experience, 90 percent of women have a sluggish metabolism, which means everything is slowed down in the body, including detox, digestion, mental firing, and weight loss to name a few. Metabolism is Step 1 on the journey to properly detox pre and especially post explant, which when addressed boosts your energy three times fold, allowing your body to heal faster.

Note: The body doesn't correct this on its own very quickly, if at all. It takes some intentional work to explore what's missing in the metabolic cycle, with mineral, metal, pathogen and hormone testing to give the body what it needs to get out of the healing crisis, usually a high alert Nervous system, adrenal/thyroid burn out, leaky gut and Histamine storms. That sounds super nerdy I know, but when you have BII, you become your own best doctor, and learn these terms, which is the silver lining in this illness, right?

Kidneys Cleansing

Water soluble toxins are eliminated by the kidneys through the urine. If the kidneys are not functioning well, other organs become overloaded with these toxins. What does a healthy urine look like? Your goal is to have odorless and colorless urine that you release around every three to four hours and not have to get up in the middle of the night to "go pee." Any more frequent is a sign your kidneys are on overdrive, which usually means you're backlogged with toxins, pathogens and/or your Central nervous system is stuck on Fight or Flight. This is why it's also important to address your mental/emotional house, because healing begins in the mind. Holding on to trapped trauma and hidden hurts from our past will keep your body in an equivalent 'holding pattern' of toxicity because 'As above, So below'.

How do you clear your kidneys? Fresh foods such as grapes, cranberries, lemons, spirulina, spinach, blueberries, nettles, dandelion, parsley, ginger, string beans, and asparagus. I suggest starting your day with a glass of warm water with fresh squeezed lemon juice with ginger and apple cider vinegar. Think you can do that instead of coffee? Check out the recipe section included at the end of this book for tonics you can try.

Blood and Lymph

The lymph and blood are the transport systems of the body. They carry nutrients to every cell as well as remove the metabolic waste products and circulate them out to the elimination channels – the colon, lungs, liver, kidneys, and skin for expulsion from the body, which is why it is important to make sure those channels are all detoxed and functioning properly first. If these systems get clogged up, you are going to get sick, implants or no implants. Supporting lymph flow and thorough blood detoxification can help. My recommendations include the following:

Castor Oil Packs: Known for improving circulation, lymphatic drainage, decreasing inflammation, and improving liver detoxification, castor oil packs are a safe, gentle, and natural way to boost your liver function. This method of detox is done by soaking an organic wool cloth in castor oil, applying it to the skin over the liver, and wearing it overnight. You'll see a lot of ways to do this on the internet, including the popular and messy approach I used to use, but I've discovered a simpler way to do this and was stoked to share with you when I heard of it. The process and products are included in my online programs, so you don't have to spend hundreds of hours I did figuring it out... Keep in mind, this is not going to chelate heavy metals out of your body, hence it is safe and gentle option for preparing for surgery to open up your detox pathways

Rebounding: Ok my all-time favorite and fun suggestion for improving the lymphatic system is to bounce around like Tigger and let your inner child party like its 1995! The way you do this is to hop on a trampoline for five to ten minutes each day. The bouncing helps pump and decongest the lymphatic fluid in the entire body. It's super simple but really effective way to support the lymphatic system.

Dry Brushing: I love dry brushing. It has been used for thousands of years to increase the circulation of blood and lymph. Bonus: it helps to smoothen the skin, reduce signs of aging and reduce the appearance of cellulite, especially in the back of the thighs.

Some additional recommendations for improving lymph flow include lymphatic massage, yoga, stretching, general exercise, and avoiding tight fitting clothes. Sorry yoga tights, it's not you, it's me! I used to live in spandex but found that when I let my skin breathe and my lymph move, my body felt better, and detox improved. My suggestion: Wear spandex sparingly...oh and Sleep naked whenever you can so your skin can breathe. Especially avoid polyester clothing because it's made of petroleum, which is a xenoestrogen and only makes your toxic burden worse, by congesting your skin with the same toxins you seek to detox from. Go for hemp, organic cotton and the like since your skin is considered your third kidney and needs to breathe!

Skin and Lungs

The skin will try to get rid of toxins that other organs fail to eliminate. If you have skin problems, look at the detox function of other organs and support them. This is the #1 root cause for acne and skin rashes, that won't resolve with topicals, nor antibiotics. It's usually your elimination systems screaming for some clearance. Here are some solutions to open these pathways, especially prior to your explant as well as post explant, while you are detoxing. These are good to practice as your regular and routine self-care rituals with the intention of self-love, otherwise what's the point, right?

Detox Baths: Sometimes detoxification can be simple and relaxing. Treat yourself to a relaxing soak in the tub. Detox baths are an excellent way to promote cleansing and can be done on a regular basis. You can assist detoxification through the skin gently by adding 1-2 cups of Epsom salts for a standard sized tub. Get non-toxic brands without fragrance or any chemical additives. This is a great way to supplement magnesium through your skin, which women are dangerously low in for many reasons, one of which is the more stressed we are in all forms, the more we use and burn out magnesium. Magnesium is a 'calming' mineral, which also offsets high levels of calcium, which is a mineral that calcifies parts of our body, such as bone. The problem however is when the body stores excess calcium (usually due to low magnesium), and it turns up as kidney, gall bladder, urinary stones like crystals that cause bladder and urinary tract infections. Supplementing magnesium with Epsom salt baths is great, however it is important to consider the sources of high calcium.

Tap water is a big one! I've studied water reports for the municipalities of the cities I support with the goal of understanding

133

their water quality and possible sources of minerals, metals and toxins like fluoride, chlorine and carcinogens they are exposed to, and let me tell you…this is where my eyes were blown wide open to how very toxic our tap water is. It's why I am emphasizing it so much right now, because our body is made up of about 55% water (60% for men) and one of the key issues in health is dehydration, which minerals regulate, hence why it's so important to detox heavy metals and to supplement with minerals.

"After having worked with thousands of clients and patients over the last decade and seeing thousands of labs, women with breast implants, struggle with similar patterns of low mineral levels, poor nutrient absorption and high heavy metal toxicity contributing to hormone and gut related disease and symptoms."

Most tap water contains high levels of calcium (hard water) which is absorbed at the highest rate in hot water, while your pores are most open. I see this often on lab tests we do in my clinic, about 80 percent of the time, revealed as 'high tissue calcium', one of the key reasons for a sluggish metabolism. **The symptoms of a sluggish metabolism are slow wound healing, depression, weight gain, stubborn belly fat, hair loss, slow hair growth, rapid aging, skin sagging, constipation and more.** And of course, a toxic body because the body can only move toxins out as rapidly as metabolism is functioning, so slow metabolism = slow detox pathways = toxic body, you see? The solution to this is to #1 have a whole house water filtration system and #2 work with a BII trained health practitioner who specializes in Functional Medicine lab testing to check your levels of Calcium, magnesium, potassium, sodium and other important minerals as well as heavy metals. To reiterate, blood testing will not reveal any of this accurately and deeply.

Deep Diaphragm Breathing not only helps eliminate waste in the form of CO_2 and brings oxygen to the tissues, but it stimulates your lymphatic system as well. **Did you know that breathing represents 70 percent of your daily detox capacity?** To get the most benefit, breathe from the diaphragm, not shallowly from the chest. Also, focus on breathing through your nose rather than your mouth. In addition to helping your body get rid of toxins, deep breathing is one of the most effective ways to reduce stress and move your Nervous system into a Parasympathetic brain state, the opposite of 'fight or flight'. This is a good thing.

Done right, breathing exercises are one of the best ways to strengthen your immune system, critical for all of us, but especially we with BII, since it's this part of your body that is responsible for warding off pathogens, detoxing chemicals and clearing hormones when the body has metabolized them. One of my favorite ways to balance my body through breathing, is alternate nostril breathing. I've been practicing and leading yoga classes and retreats for the last 2 decades, and this is my favorite way to start class, and a powerful tool you can use throughout the day anytime you feel a stress response mounting in your body...you know...when your kids are going cray, your partner is acting a fool or your inner b*tch just won't leave you TF alone!

"Just 30 minutes of daily meditation and intentional breath work can lower anxiety and depression levels up to 38%—about the same amount as an antidepressant."

Why alternate nostril breathing? Your nose is directly linked to your brain and nervous system. For thousands of years the Indian yogis believe that most diseases are connected to disturbed nasal breathing.

Breathing in through your left nostril will access the right "feeling" hemisphere of your brain, and breathing in through your right nostril, will access the left "thinking" hemisphere of your brain. Consciously alternating your breath between either nostril will allow you to activate and access your whole brain.

Step one: Use right thumb to close off right nostril.

Step two: Inhale slowly through left nostril

Step three: Pause for a second

Step four: Now close left nostril with ring finger and release thumb off right nostril

Step five: Exhale through your right nostril

Step six: Now, inhale through right nostril

Step seven: Pause

Step eight: Use thumb to close of right nostril

Step nine: Breathe out through left nostril

Step ten: This is one round. Start slowly with 1 or 2 rounds and gradually increase. Never force. Sit quietly for a few moments after you have finished.

This is just one technique I like and use. There are many, many different techniques of pranayama such as inhaling for 4, holding for 4 and exhaling for 4, that you can do 10 times for a quick chill break. Wim Hof is the master of breath work, I recommend checking him out too.

Double down your results and pleasure your senses by doing this with your favorite essential oils. Eucalyptus is great to expand your lungs, orange is a mood booster and lavender calms your mind, so let your intuition guide you to suit your needs.

Sweating: Working up a sweat is hands own the most effective and easiest way to support your body's natural ability to detox. You can do this through exercise pre-explant, but post-explant I highly recommend sitting in an infrared sauna as tolerated 3-4 times per week for 30-60 minute sessions. I have an entire protocol for this in my online programs involving all of these techniques to simplify your detox journey by stacking your hacks'. It is not only incredibly relaxing and calms your Central nervous system, reducing the fight or flight state most of us are stuck in especially with BII, but has amazing detoxification and healing benefits.

For the average human today, 70% of our day we operate in a fight or flight, stressed response from a mental / emotional perspective. Add to that the toxins from breast implants, toxic beauty and toxins all around us, and it's no wonder so many of us with breast implants struggle to cope with stress, let alone make it through the day. When the limbic system of your brain is working to protect yourself from a major threat externally, it's unable to protect you from a major threat internally, such as a virus.

If you have HPA-axis dysfunction (confirmed by proper Functional medicine lab testing), you should only do this with the guidance of a qualified health practitioner. Reach out to me if you would like support with this. Additionally, I also highly advise having your own sauna at home, preferably a Full Spectrum unit Before you buy one, I recommend you check out the videos in my programs and in the Resources section because the majority are toxic, made with cheap materials, made in China, exclude your head or are loaded with EMF's, adding further stress to the body! Hot tip for perspective: Good Saunas start at between $3-5,000 so if you're spending less than that, it's probably toxic AF, and in that case it's not 'better than nothing' because you're adding toxins back into your body, which is the goal of sitting in a sauna to begin with right?

If we truly learn our lesson from BII, it's to research exactly what is contained in the things we use in, on and around our body and not blindly trust...or if you don't want to take the time to, and would rather trust someone who has done the research for you, that's what I've done and those are the solutions I provide to you.

Anything I recommend and stand behind, are things I have researched, and tried or own myself.

All of these detox techniques will vary for each woman on her way to explant and beyond. They are all generally safe and effective, but every person will respond differently. There's a lot of contradictory information you will find on what is 'safe with implants' or not, but it's too hard to say unless you're working 1 on 1 with a BII trained practitioner who knows your medical history, labs and lifestyle. For example, what I learned in doing the heaps of research I did on BII, Botox is more dangerous for many women than breast implants and can have extremely distressful side effects for women who deep detox within the first 4 weeks post injection. This is why it's important to consider all aspects of your life before attempting explant, detox and healing in general.

Over time, once you progressively rid your body of these toxins and heal your tissues, I recommend maintaining these strategies as a part of your routine, even after you have fully recovered from BII.

Pre-Explant checklist

Since you'll be a little out of commission for 4 weeks or so, you'll want to prepare things ahead of time to ensure a smooth transition. Here's a list of things to consider:

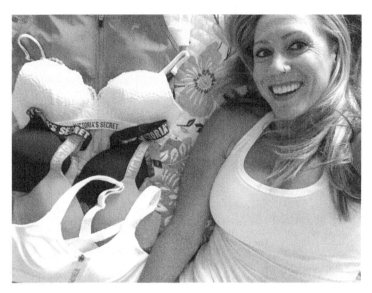

I bought 5 new bras to welcome in my new boobies

- Buy new bras. Talk with your doctor about the proper sizes for ones you will transition into after your surgery bra.

- Buy two 'surgery' bras, so you always have a clean one, while you can't do laundry. Get a zip front, compression type bra that doesn't choke you or cut off your circulation too much, like I did. I ordered mine online which was the right size, but it was really small, but it was too late by the time I found out. Bring yours to your pre-op appointment to get the thumbs up from your surgeon, especially because you don't want one that is too tight, since it will push against your drains and hurt like hell.

- Buy compression undergarments if you are doing fat transfer. Your doctor will help you pick them out, as the styles are always changing, but essentially, it's like wearing tight Spanx that compress on the areas where you had lipo.

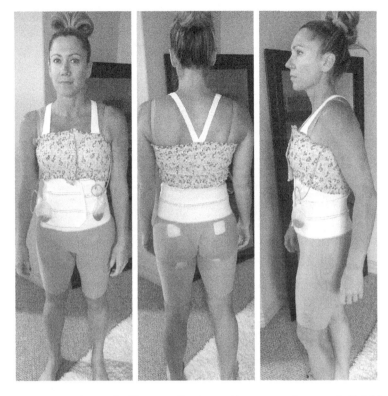

Check out my hot outfit. This is my Tinder profile pic now, drains and all. LOL

- Do all your laundry, dishes, have the house clean, a few days prior. Set out comfy clothes and wear baggy, comfy's the day of your surgery.
- Tell work you need at least two weeks off, maybe four.
- Have all your meds and supplements ready to go and organized for the person who is caring for you.

- Have a relative come stay with you for seven days at least, ten days if you have fat transfer just in case. I was able to drive after that as most women are.

- Buy healing groceries prior to. Make tons of soups and broths. Pre-made green juices, ACV with lemon, kombucha, sole was super helpful for my mom just to pour into a glass and throw a stainless-steel straw into.

- Have soul food ready. You can pick from a good book, documentaries, funny movies and uplifting shows, but I highly recommend against just binging on Netflix, because this is your time to create your rebuilding plan. I'm a little impartial, but if I were you I would check out that online program, the Warrior Cleanse and watch those videos or CHI, where you can watch videos and have Diane on speed dial in case you need her or her team during this time. Hee-hee!

- Definitely bring a sloth with you to the surgery. You need a reminder to smile through it all, be patient with yourself, fear nothing and slow the F down. Trust me, it will cheer you up!

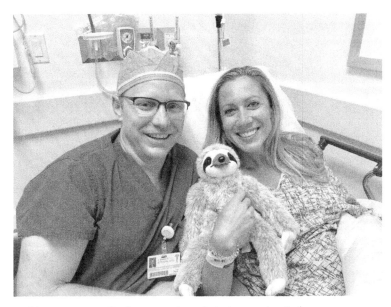

Me, my surgeon, Dr Strawn and my sloth the morning before my surgery

What Should I Expect pre and post explant?

Hang on for the ride, let's get your expectations hat on first.

This isn't a walk in the park, as simple as just cutting these "toxic tit bags" out and getting back to work the next day. Although, I certainly had moments where I walked up to my friends with a steak knife and gestured toward my breasts and asked, "Will you do the honors?" ... when they eye rolled and laughed at me, I followed with a "C'mon, I'll let you grab my boobs."

A *huge* part of this journey is learning to laugh and not take yourself so damn seriously. For real.

Hypervigilance.

Anger.

Betrayal.

These are all emotions along the spectrum we *all* experience, so know you're not alone. This is totally normal, *but* you don't have to bathe in it. And although you will be tested and feel like you're on your last leg of patience, it's not a hall pass to be a royal b*tch to the people in your life, including yourself!

I'll help you with some coping and emotional freedom/calming techniques in the 'Ignite' Chapter of this book, but for now, let's get back to "what to expect" so you can focus the little bits of energy you have on getting your body ready for this exorcism we call explant, and also maybe things that are food for your soul like hanging with your kids, or having rocking sex with your partner... That is if your hormones are still on board and you're not living in hell with UTI's, chronic yeast and or interstitial cystitis - all common BII symptoms and conditions I myself and our clients experienced recovering from BII. Thankfully, the chances of those things disappearing soon, if you follow the recommendations in this book to the tee, will be high.

It's important for you to know the things that most don't brace themselves well enough for. I certainly didn't when I began my BII journey:

- Detox takes *work*
- Healing takes *time*
- Emotional mastery takes *patience*

Every woman should work for at least one-year post explant to restore her gut, hormones, brain chemicals, and heart/mindset while also detoxing chemicals and metals from her body.

For example, your body rebuilds itself in one year, overall with the brain taking the longest (1 year), then the blood (4 months), bones (3 months), DNA (2 months), Liver (6 weeks), skin (1 month), lungs (2-3 weeks) and stomach (5 days).

And this is a normal human without implants.

When you add this level of toxicity to the mix and you gum up the irrigation pipes, many of us need two or three years of concentrated, customized and loving focus on recovering our bodies. That is, unless you want to roll the dice in paying the price later with worsening diseases, usually in your family history's weakest genetic link – cancer, auto immune disease, heart attack, stroke, and mood-related disease being the highest, by JUST removing your implants, which many women do, but oftentimes experience many symptoms and disease because they didn't customize a plan to suit their body and the damage their implants caused

Special note to women who are aspiring to have children now or at a later date. Please give your body at *least* six months of customized cleansing, healing your gut/hormones, and igniting your life post explant, otherwise you are more likely to dump toxins from your breast implants into your baby and perpetuate the cycle for generations beyond.

Chapter 6: Soul Goal – If You Want to Fly, You Must Know Your Why

This is a powerful journey you are on. It's very important to journal your journey, share with others, be open, vulnerable and practice speaking your voice authentically realizing that the only judgment you are feeling is the one judging you in your head. This is the voice that drove us to get implants in the first place, right?

What I've noticed in my experience working with women for ten years in this industry, is this: If your dream isn't bigger than your nightmare, you won't get better. If you don't have a target, you will miss it every time. Without a *soul goal*, you are like a ship at sea with no sails. You bounce around like a skipping rock across the ocean, subject to the storms at sea. Your life purpose, what I refer to as your soul goal is the *deepest* divinity of who you came here to be and what you came here to do.

You have suffered. Remember when you were "going through it" ... You wished there was someone you could turn to for support? Often times for many, this becomes their gift. They walked through darkness, adversity, and the most difficult of times, got through it and thought ... "Now I wish to help others and provide the support I was looking for when this all went down."

A great consideration for your soul goal is by asking the younger you: If I could give my X-year-old advice, what would I have to say to her? Prior to the trauma and challenging times. Many find this is the kind of work they wish to birth into the world to help others who are lost

In the midst of the pity parties, inner child fits and drama cycles we women all go through, it helps distract you from the pain of your experience, by focusing on love, which also spikes a hormone called Oxytocin in the body, one of the most powerful anti-inflammatory's, stress suppressants and feel good hormones, that the majority of us are dangerously low in today. Especially we with breast implants. How can our hearts connect physically to one another in an embrace when we have gigantic sacks of fake toxins blocking us? I don't have any science to prove this, but my suspicion is that, the amount of chemicals would be reduced, especially in breastfeeding women, who in my clinical experience tend to have babies with more issues at birth and beyond, such as: compromised immunity, allergies, EMF/radiation and food/chemical sensitivities, learning disorders, bowel and skin issues and more.

In fact, part of my soul goal is to spread this message to women, aspiring mothers who struggle to get pregnant and breastfeed because my long list of kid clients are those with the aforementioned symptoms including seizures, auto immune disease, and Autism just to name a few. I have been approached by many women who see the work I am doing, what I am up to in the world, mainly in the realms of loving ourselves as we are, living unapologetically us, learning the art of self-care and listening to our bodies innate wisdom through intuition and they approach me and say: "What you are doing is my Soul Goal...how can I help others by teaching the same"? My answer: I teach warrior woman to be loving leaders through my Warrior Coach Certification program. You can find all of that info in the Resources section on my website.

You might find yourself, like many, asking 'What's my Purpose'? And then if you're like most women I work with, they stress out about trying to 'figure it out'. News flash: If you're using your brain to force an answer, it won't be an authentic answer. If you ask your heart questions with the intention of discovering truths from the wise woman, the strong warrior and the wounded child, you are much more likely to find the answer. Here's the formula I created that has helped many of my clients:

Ask yourself:

- What are you most *passionate* about teaching?

- What are you most *angry* about in the world you wish would cease to exist?

- What are you *curious* about learning?

- What medicine do *you* most need to hear?

- What *gifts* do you believe are unique to you, which you wish to share?

- What thing or things do you have the most *wisdom* around you feel confident helping others with?

- Once you have crafted your soul goal draft 1 or revision, ask yourself:

- What are the three reasons why you deserve this?

Then...

- What are the three reasons others deserve you expressing your soul goal?

"A soul goal is something you *want* to give to the world, to others, something you want to do every day, embodying all things. Empathy, wisdom and creativity ... Such that it gets you out of bed in the morning and gives you more energy than every stimulant in the world ... Where coffee doesn't work, and where life throws you off course ... Your *soul goal* pops in to vitalize you, revive you, and remind you of the mission you're on and the heart work you came here to do."

It doesn't have to be about suffering either, although often times this is the inner work we seek deep down. It could be fun, upbeat, anything that makes you *come alive*.

In its simplest form I've boiled it down to this: Somewhere between what you're good at, what you care about, and what you are deeply passionate (angry) about ... You will discover your *soul goal*.

If you discovered tomorrow was your last day on this Earth, have you sung the song you came here to sing? What regret would you have? What one thing do you wish you would have spoken up about that will die when you do, yet with one day left, it has the chance to live, by passing it onto others, who will carry the torch? And most importantly: What struggle or sacrifice are you willing to endure? Because in the end, it's not those who simply seek out their soul goal and they nail it first try, it's those who continue on over and over, without losing their enthusiasm. That is success.

And once you have this down, it will drive you to places you wouldn't have thought possible, pull you when you run out of energy, provide clarity where there was once fog. Life will make a lot more sense to you.

And in the meantime, until you have your purpose ... Do everything in your life *on* purpose, with all your heart. Enjoy every moment and wake up every day with gratitude, celebrating your wins *and* your fails at the end of the day... Because they taught you something too (like your breast implants).

The greatest way to receive love is to give love. And the greatest way to learn something is to master the art of teaching it. How do you think I learned how to write this book to help you? I surrendered fully into the pain of it, to find my purpose in it. It made the journey a hellofa lot easier, knowing that there was a reason for my lessons, and that was to learn the art of loving myself the way I am, to not blindly trust and to learn how to listen to my body so I can teach you to do the same. To me, when I think about it, a learned lesson not shared, is a wasted experience. Wisdom is meant to be handed down to fellow humans and future generations.

Along my path to release the hold of the pain I held in my body that lead me to cut myself open, ashamed of who I was, wanting to be something I was not, I found myself in a ceremonial meditation where I broke through and broke free from a trauma

150

wound that was fueling my inner b*tch, bully voice that told me I wasn't beautiful and whole as I was. These are the ceremonies I organize and host for women to help them heal in tranquil places like Costa Rica, Greece, Punta Cana, Hawaii and Sedona.

PHOENIX RISING

Last nights sacred gathering revealed the most powerful vision I have ever seen and felt.

I asked my guides for Clarity, Compassion, Connection and Consciousness to honor the voice inside of me that said:

One day a wise voice in my head gently whispered

Do not remove your **Breast Implants** until you've learned the Lesson you bought them to teach you.

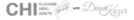

I knew it was going to be a Powerful journey...

I was being pulled apart like Slink from Toy Story...only I was balls of matter, not a slinky.

Balls of Matter.

Reminding me how much I matter.

My journey matters.

Your journey matters.

We do not stumble upon suffering by accident.

It is by design.

For us to wake up.

In my vision...I got to see, like never before...where I was trapped in my own

body.

Chakras imprisoned by my programming.

Conditioning.

Culture.

Schooling.

Jail Cell.

Cell death.

Cell phone dependence.

Caged.

The illusion of freedom.

The seduction of sovereignty.

The lies I believed that…

In order to get the Dream Life I "should" want, I needed to shape my body

like Barbie.

The half-naked women in rap videos 36-24-36...but only if she's 5'3".

They were the ones getting attention in the videos, ads, movies.

They get the most likes on Instagram.

They are the most popular.

Fake tits.

Yep that's the answer.

To be a sell out to my own body, in exchange to (jail) 'cell in' my heart

chakra.

Block my heart with the prison cells shaped as silicone breast implants.

My vision revealed barbed wire around my implants.

Barbed wire?

Barbie.

Barbie wire?

Body dysmorphia, eating disorders, retail 'therapy'?

Ouuccchhhh...it hurt so bad to feel the prison of programming.

For me, for all women, for us all, for my ancestors.

I felt stabbing pains and shocks through my heart, lungs and chest cavity.

Rapid heartbeat, trying to break through the landmines of toxicity on top of

them

Passion rising through the pain.

Purpose piercing plasticity.

PHOENIX RISING from her Ashes.

INTENSE feelings connecting to the Universe, Mother and all that is.

It was the first time I needed to ask for help during ceremony.

My Shaman sang to me, extracted the pain, the programming, the prison.

My soul sisters raced over to wrap me with their wings

Embraced me with love.

When my soul sister Alicia Marie, placed her hand on my heart, I felt the beat

of my abandoned soul return home.

She felt safe to return.

A nest of radical self-love and acceptance.

It brings me to tears of joy and love reliving this as I type…

Because I have lived so much of my life sold out to my soul.

Soul out. Sell out. Cell out. Out of body.

What's it all for?

Now I know.

Return to love.

Soul in.

In flow.

In love.

In joy.

Enjoy.

The next vision, I was sitting with my mom on the rim of a garden.

I was a young girl.

She had her arm around me, and I was crying.

A baby deer came fourth and said to my mom 'Is the little girl sad? Why is she crying?'

And in that moment, I lost it.

Through the purge of my tears, I lost the story.

I dropped the shame.

The guilt.

The race to 'fit in'.

To matter.

To do.

Months later, now I feel, what was revealed, that part of me healed.

Deer is heart medicine.

The visions orchestrated just for me.

For my highest.

So I can climb out of this cell.

To restore my cells.

To let out what does not serve.

And to let in what does.

In 5 days, I explant.

It is not just removing tox-SICK silicone bags from my body.

It is the removal of my old self, programmed to speak 'not enough' into my subconscious.

Friday morning, I get out of prison.

Get out of Jail free? NO.

It came with a price.

It cost me my health.

But what I gained was self-wealth.

And a love for myself, I have never felt before.

Out with the silicone, in with the soul.

I am BEYOND grateful for all of my friends, family, teachers and for Spirit guiding me through this journey.

I pushed people away so I could bring ME back in.

The me I disowned years ago.

It has been tumultuous yet transformative.

It is preparing me for something huge, and I am humbled Spirit chose me to fight this fire, so I could help others.

I have been CHOSEN to walk through hell so I could walk out of the flames stronger, carrying buckets of water for those still consumed by the fire.

From Pain to Purpose.

May we all take the Call and have the Courage to Hear the Message.

 AHO

To me, this is the most important part of the pre-explant journey. Get essential oils to activate your senses, calm your mind, open your heart and heal your body. Forgive yourself for making the choice that rendered you sick. Sometimes, it's guilt that can make us sicker than the implants themselves. This is a topic for a whole other book, and a big part of the one on one work I do with clients, so for now, remember to be gentle with you knowing you are doing and have always done your best, from your level of thinking. And now you are learning better choices and upgrading your thinking in a major way!

What a gift, this powerful lesson you are learning, sister!

Chapter 7: Cleanse - Time to Go Deep, Your Crucial Step Number 1

At this point in the game, you will have explanted. YAY for you. First, give yourself a lot of credit and kudos for taking this huge step. Your body thanks you in advance, even though it may not feel like it yet, since you're probably numbed out on a lot of good meds.

My goal for you in this chapter is to learn the right way to cleanse for you and for a woman with a history of BII. If you get this wrong, it will be a waste (pun intended).

The top three myths I hear on the regular about detox post explant are these:

- Myth: Every symptom I have after explant is a result of detox reaction.

Truth: Breast Implants and most surgical devices cause our bodies a tremendous amount of stress and destruction that require deeper healing than simply removing the source. Symptoms are rarely detox-oriented, but more so signs of something still unwell and unhealed post explant. Detox should not cause unwanted symptoms, misery, or debilitation.

- Myth: My body can't detox because I have the MTHFR genetic mutation, so I'm screwed.

Truth: Your genetics can be overridden by your lifestyle, toxic exposure, supplements, stress levels, diet, beliefs and thoughts.

- Myth: Chlorella, cilantro, and spirulina are good binders for detox post explant surgery.

- Truth: They are very weak bonds and can cause more harm with women who carry a heavy metal load from having breast implants. Stronger detox bonds are highly imperative!

By now you already know breast implants are *super* toxic and they impact every woman who has them... And come to think about it, *every* person who has any implant. Now when you think about our environment today, and add to that stress, plus breast implants and other medical devices that wear out our immune systems, it seems pretty apparent why so many of us struggle with excess fat, fatigue and frustration, disease, depression, and death.

"Since World War Two, 80,000 new chemicals have been created, and to add to that, a whopping 1,500 new ones each year. One would assume that someone is out there regulating all this stuff, but testing is next to nothing: approximately ten of these 1,500 chemicals will be tested for their neurotoxic effect and zero will be tested to explore reactions with other chemicals that have been approved, something called the synergist effect, which can have thousands of unique reactions and side effects when combined and ingested."

You ever read "proprietary formula" on the label of cleaning chemicals? This means 'we're not telling you what toxins are in this'. How can they get away with this lack of transparency? The reason why is because they are protected by trade secrets, hence many companies are not legally obligated to disclose their ingredients. Worse, they are consciously including carcinogenic (cancer-causing) ingredients proven to cause neurotoxic (brain disruptive) effects, with no ramifications. Does this piss you off as much as it does me? The literal causes for disease today are heavily marketed to us as convenient concoctions, yet the rule of thumb seems to be:

"The more you see products marketed on TV, in magazines or are household names, the more toxic they are. A fun slogan I say is 'If it's on TV, it's not good for me'. The good news is, natural and safe is making a comeback, but it's not mainstream so let this book guide you in the right direction and if you're confused about your Soul Goal, perhaps you can jump on this Transparency Train to teach others how to live clean lives. We need more people teaching these solutions."

Unfortunately, most are mistaken and misled on how to do a comprehensive cleanse in the right order and deeply enough, especially us who have explanted and have BII. Our cleanse approach is completely unique for reasons we already went over in previous chapters.

There are two things you must consider with a cleanse and that is this:

- You must cleanse *inside* of your body,
- Cleanse the toxins around you that add to your toxic load.

Many of those I have already mentioned under "Preparing for Explant" on cleaning up your diet and will also cover in future chapters on swapping out toxic beauty, home, cleaning cosmetics, and personal care products in your home. Because what good would it do to do all this work to cleanse your body while at the same time giving it even *more* work to slather toxic chemicals all over it? Remember:

"Everything you add to your skin, your body must work hard to digest and detox within".

This chapter will focus more on how to cleanse your body both from the toxins you have absorbed prior to conception and throughout your whole life plus the residue of the implants. But first ... Let's make sure you don't waste your time, money, and energy on these super common cleanse fails.

Here are the ten main fails I see people run into with cleansing that not only don't work, they actually can make things worse:

1. Not addressing the mind-body connection
2. Using cheap or toxic cleanse supplements
3. Not using powerful binders and detox strategies to carry toxins out of the body
4. Not consuming cleansing foods that support detox
5. Cleansing during a stressful time
6. Cleansing while not getting proper rest
7. Cleansing without proper hydration

8. Incomplete cleanses that miss organs, or address them in the wrong order

9. Cleansing without simultaneously opening eliminatory pathways

10. Not cleansing for long enough, or finishing but going back to the unhealthy lifestyle that created the need to cleanse in the first place

If you get these wrong, cleansing can take longer, make you want to give up, and cause you to slip back into your old ways, thinking that there's no hope for you. Change takes time, but the progress you make toward positive, lasting change can slip away in a fraction of that time, if you do it the wrong way and don't address each one of these in detail:

#1 Not Addressing the Mind-Body Connection

You'll learn more about this in the 'Ignite' chapter, mainly how to handle stress, to simplify your life and how to change your mind by changing how you see the world.

"Life is 10 percent what happens to you and 90 percent how you respond to it."

If you respond to stress with more stress, you'll create more acidity inside of the body, drain your hormones, stall detox pathways, and wonder why it didn't work.

#2 Using Cheap or Toxic Cleanse Supplements

The supplement industry is *highly* unregulated. They can say whatever they want on labels and get away with it-- promising you the moon, even though you'll feel more like Uranus (LOL). The thing is, over 90% of supplements are full of the very toxins you are looking to clear from the body, so it's *imperative* to use supplements that have been tested for heavy metal levels, don't have folic acid in them (terrible for MTHFR genes – you want methylfolate), and/or have toxic fillers and binders. Most supplements are absorbed 10 percent at best, while the remaining 90 percent are excreted from the body. Add to that a leaky gut with compromised nutrient absorption, common to we with BII, and you have 'expensive urine'. Your hard-earned dollar flushed down the toilet, literally!

So, then what's the point, right? The reason the ones I use with my client's work is because they go to great lengths to ensure all of these prerequisites are met. *Hint:* If it's sold at CVS or if it's sold at a store, chances are it's not powerful or high quality enough for you post explant because the doses are so low. In fact, I created an entire line to suit the needs of women suffering from Toxic Beauty symptoms, because it didn't exist, so I made it happen! Call it my 'Soul Goal' in a bottle.

#3 Not Using Powerful Binders and Detox Strategies to Carry Toxins out of the Body

There are a few binders that are powerful enough to carry toxins out of the body. Fulvic acid, humic acid, activated charcoal, pectins, zeolites, and EDTA. Unfortunately, I see *so many* women who have been recommended to take Chlorella, cilantro, and spirulina as good binders for detox post explant surgery. The truth is, they are very weak bonds and can cause more harm for women who carry a heavy metal load from having breast implants, because they may pull the toxins from a safer place like fat cells, but because they initiate such a weak bond, they usually drop them before they leave the body, rendering them in a *more* toxic form than before. Also, worth mentioning is that not all zeolites are treated alike. There are loads of companies that claim to have high levels of ingredients, only to have been tested for a fraction of what they claim. My friends, do not be fooled by glitter marketing and sorry to say but most Multi-Level Marketing companies are known to hype up testimonies. I have been a part of many and have witnessed the behind the scenes representatives who parrot the advisory board educators, but have no experience of their own with clients, nor are health practitioners, so buyer beware!

When it comes to 'kick ass binders' for detox, look for a blend that is multi-faceted. There are a few I like to use with clients, selected intentionally so you don't have to take ten different supplements for ten different things. It covers a lot of ground like, binding to bio-toxins (candida, molds, etc.) in the intestines, plus clears viruses and prevents reabsorption as it absorbs up to 300 times its weight in toxins. Stronger detox bonds are highly imperative. And I'll say one last thing here. When I started my BII journey and googled "best supplements to cleanse post explant" what came up was a long confusing ass list of over 100 plus supplements without any mention of how long to take them and when. I wanted to quit before I even started, and I knew if I felt that way as a practitioner, so would you. This was a huge inspiration for me to write this book, so I could simplify things for you! If you're like me and 'just want to be told what to do' without having to do a ton of research, I put the brand and blends I like the most in the 'Resources' section of my website.

#4 Not Consuming Cleansing Foods That Support Detox

You just can't expect to eat junk food and cleanse at the same time and get results. It's crucial you consume healthy foods, such as fat, to gobble up and carry out fat soluble toxins through the bowels, and fiber plus DIM rich foods such as kale, collard, broccoli and cauliflower to sweep up and carry out toxins through the bowels, especially xenoestrogens. If you want to learn how to do this and create systems around it, making it realistic, fun and customized to you, check out my Warrior Cleanse, an online program that teaches you everything you need to know and excludes everything you didn't about how to eat to love on your liver, hormones, gut and entire body!

#5 Cleansing During a Stressful Time

I mean, we're kind of always stressed out today. It seems crazy busy is the trend, right? But let's just say this. If you're going through a *major* life change and you can barely get out of bed, this is a case-by-case situation where you should absolutely consult a practitioner who has experience, education and empathy with women suffering with BII, and can help you with calming your stress load, activating your metabolic pathways, and getting your hormones on board for energy, before the detox.

#6 Cleansing While Not Getting Proper Rest

98 percent of fat burning happens at night, and detox takes a lot of work. Melatonin is a major inflammatory hormone so if you're not getting at least seven to nine hours of sleep at the proper circadian rhythm between 10 p.m. and 6 a.m., you're not resting optimally. Oh, and side note: This sleep hormone has also been said to be instrumental in protecting us from Viruses such as CV-19. More on sleep in Chapter 12.

#7 Cleansing without Proper Hydration

Many toxins are water soluble, so they can't leave the body without the bodyguard to escort it out, namely *water*. Also, be sure it's properly *filtered* water as well. Reminder: Brita, Pur, and Bottled water are not even close to meeting this, unless it's Essentia that's pretty much the only water I buy if I'm in a pinch and don't have any. I list the current water filtration companies I love and use myself in the Resources section of my website.

#8 Incomplete Cleanses That 'Miss' Organs, or Address Them in the Wrong Order

Epic fail when it comes to cleansing. I see it all the time! Imagine a kitchen sink that is clogged…what happens when you turn on the water? It spills out right? Then you have a mess everywhere. On the same token, before you start dislodging toxins from their hiding places, it's imperative that you do 3 things, this is the 3B jumpstart: Boost metabolism, balance hormones and bowel cleansing. This gives you the proper energy, balanced throughout the day to jumpstart and sustain the power it takes to detox, and opens up the main pathway to clear them. Remember detox takes work and it takes an exit strategy. I'll get more detailed about how to do this in the 'Heal' chapter.

#9 Not cleansing for long enough, or finishing, but going back to the unhealthy lifestyle that created the need to cleanse in the first place.

In three days or even a month or three, you can't expect to clear twenty to thirty years' worth of low-level heavy metal toxicity, which as you have already read, takes *at least* one year to cleanse and that's assuming you *don't* have a history of implants. You can

166

two or three X that for we who have had implants. Hence, patience, a plan, and persistence are required to do this right. That may sound like a long time but consider the alternatives. If they *don't* get cleared out properly now, it will mean higher odds of symptoms and suffering later. And, you know what type of woman I see most? One who has spent $50,000-60,000+ on the doctor, guru, naturopath treadmill on protocols that mostly or only treat the lab results but not the lifestyle that created them. Do you want to spend that much, or do you want to spend 1/10 of that doing it right the first time?

#10 Cleansing Without Simultaneously Opening Up Eliminatory Pathways

As I mentioned in #8 above, your colon needs to be an open door, available to release toxins from your body, otherwise they will U turn back into your body, causing more damage. It's like puking in your mouth and swallowing it. I know that's a disgusting visual but it's important for you to digest just how important this is. You can say the same thing about your skin. Someone who doesn't sweat is akin to not pooping for weeks at a time. Imagine if your garbage man forgot to come for months, how many maggots, flys, bugs and stench would emit from your trash bin. Then bacteria comes around to break down the fermented food and waste and animals swarm to eat the bacteria, which is exactly what happens in your body.

Your body is that intelligent that it will create bugs to break down food and toxins you are unable to release yourself. This is a huge reason today most of us are loaded with bad bugs, yet doctors best solution is anti-biotics, which further worsen your gut microbes, because they kill the good bugs too, which give you immunity, beauty and energy. So, the answer is not to go on a candida, parasite, bacteria killing spree, which is what I see many women do, mistakenly mislead by their practitioners or incomplete advice online. The answer is to explore why the bugs are there to begin with, explore detox and digestion pathways and optimize the big picture so everything is working together.

I don't know about you, but when I learned this, my heart cracked wide open and I dropped down to my knees in tears of gratitude in awe at just how intelligent our body and Creator is. I apologized to myself for never thanking it for always looking out for me, protecting me and self-regulating to try to get my attention with symptoms. This continued through my journey to explant when I discovered lumps in my breasts, my ribs continually went out and my bowels released silicone.

Your body is always on guard to love you, liberate you and save your life. This is where I learned empathy for myself and others and is why it's critical to work with someone who has been through this. It's truly a spiritual journey that opens your third eye, your mind and your heart.

To sum it up, this is where it helps immensely to enlist the support of a qualified practitioner who has three things to amplify your odds of success: empathy, education, and experience.

Let's dive into the 3 E's applied to the intricate order for deep cleansing.

Step 1: The Five-R Protocol for Cellular Detox

One of my mentors Dr. Dan Pompa says, "In order to get well, you must fix the cell". And the hot topic on the streets now is 'Mending the Mitochondria' which is to say fixing the body at the most micro level by taking the cells through a Cleanse, Heal, Ignite process. This process is where you begin supporting the cell function (via the 5R's). It should take one to three months, depending on the person, and relies on the following: how much toxicity they have in the body, how healthy they were functioning before they started their cleanse phase, and how consistent they are. For example, if you have a ton of oral infections, cavitations, and/or root canals that remain post explant, or if you decide to keep your breast implants, you won't be able to fix the cells at their core, because the source of the toxins are still living in your body. It's important to address or remove those before you can move into the deeper phases of cleansing. Note that if you don't, you will have to spend more to detox, making healing more difficult. Take it from me who spent $100,000+ on trying to heal my body with the ticking time bombs still living inside of me.

With this BII approach, when starting a cleanse, you use the 5R's as the roadmap and these principles remain the foundation throughout our approach to fixing the cell. This is a clinically proven strategy that has helped thousands earn their lives back, after mainstream medicine has failed them. The process is not a quick-fix band-aid but rather a guide for you to understand how to support all of your health challenges. The following steps are often addressed simultaneously, but it depends upon the case, as the goal is not to focus on a specific condition, but to fully support the body's inherent ability to heal itself. Here they are in order:

R1: Remove the Source

Our protocol begins by determining which sources of stress are causing body-wide damage and removing them as soon as possible. R1 is removing the toxic source that has accumulated over time in the body. It's nearly impossible to recover health without removing major sources of toxicity such as breast implants or mercury amalgam fillings (but removal *must* be performed properly, or detox becomes dangerous). Most allopathic doctors cover-up symptoms with medications while, alternative practitioners often do the same, except with supplements. Neither approach gets people truly well. Getting "knee-to-knee" with you and digging deep into your health history (including physical, emotional and chemical stressors) is key to figuring out what caused the sickness Toxins quickly shut down detox pathways and allow other toxins to bio-accumulate. In women with breast implants, this includes biotoxins (from mold and Lyme disease), infections and heavy metals, such as

170

lead and mercury. To keep it simple, I call it the 3 M's: Mycotoxins, microbes and metals.

R2: Regenerate the Cell Membrane

Your cell membranes hold the intelligence of the cell, and it plays a major role in detoxification, as well as turning genes off & on, and regulating hormones. Regenerating the membrane is at the core of solving a growing number of unexplainable symptoms and degenerative diseases seen all too often today at epidemic proportions. In healthy individuals, the supple lipid bilayer of the membrane allows nutrients, hormones, minerals to flow inside easily, while toxins and free radicals get rejected. If inflamed, the cell door closes, and the nutrients can't get in, nor can the toxins leave, so the cell becomes a toxic wasteland, resulting in symptoms, sickness and suffering. In order to properly clear toxins and absorb nutrients, the membrane must be regenerated.

Remember when I mentioned 'expensive urine'? When you fix the cell, it can receive the vitamins you buy that you work so hard for. And hormones too...one of the big fails I see with clients who come to me on Thyroid medication and taking Exogenous hormones like HRT and bio identicals is that their doctor prescribed them without considering the health of the cell and detox potential of the liver and colon. Whatever you are not absorbing, gets recycled if you are not properly detoxing it, which most aren't. When this happens, these hormones simply recycle and cause things

171

like heart palpitations in the case of thyroid mediations, and tissue growths such as fibroids, cancer, fat cells, cysts, tumors in the case of women taking exogenous estrogen and progesterone.

"Whatever doesn't get into the cell, can quite literally make you feel like hell!".

R3: Restore Cellular Energy

Cellular energy is the fuel and fire of the cell, and nothing runs or functions without it. When nutrients enter your cell, they feed mitochondria, the mighty energy makers that produce ATP (cellular energy). Without adequate production of ATP, your cells can't detox or regenerate optimally (R1 and R2). I am a great example of this, as a pro athlete who always had low ATP...the lower your ATP, the more inflammation occurs at the cellular level.

Being low on ATP is not just an issue with women who have BII, it's become a major epidemic in America. The less energy your cells make, the less energy you have, are you with me? Clients who have come to me with chronic fatigue, irresponsibly diagnosed with 'adrenal fatigue' (which doesn't exist), brain fog, belly bloat, digestive challenges and hormone imbalances have all tried what feels like everything, with every practitioner and done every lab. Yet what most of them have not tried is to raise cellular ATP and fix the cell. Without the 5R protocol, all the treatments in the world won't fix the symptoms...for the long run at least!

R4: Reduce Cellular Inflammation

Systemic cellular inflammation is driving the epidemic of hormone conditions and the chronic diseases which are so pervasive in our culture today, especially in toxic beauty and BII. Specifically, in reference to inflammation of the cell membrane, affecting the way the cell communicates, detoxes and ultimately changes gene expression, potentially triggering a disease of genetic weakness Genetic mutations create an environment that makes us more susceptible to advanced illness, like cancer and auto immune disease. Understanding how inflammation affects the cell, and how to downregulate it, is essential to healing almost any condition.

Unfortunately, most health practitioners are not up to date with the exciting research in the area of inflammation, detox, or gene expression, nor are taught how to fix cells at the root in this way in medical school. If they did, and they recommended it to you, your results would have been radically improved, quickly... The main sources for inflammation are breast implants, Botox, toxic beauty ingredients, dietary sugars and grains, PUFA's (inflammatory fats like vegetable and canola oil), biotoxins, toxins from mercury fillings, vaccines, GMOs and others. I teach you how to avoid all of these in detail and in steps, in my online program, The Warrior Cleanse.

R5: Re-Establish Methylation

Methylation is a term you definitely want to know. It's basically SuperDetox that occurs from your inner Detox Diva's, including DNA repair, detoxification, fighting infections, removing environmental toxins (such as lead and estrogen mimicking chemicals) as well as more processes we're only beginning to understand. The body needs methylation to regulate stress hormones, and when we're unable to methylate, our bodies remain in a state of constant stress. Are you starting to get the many reasons your body is in 'fight or flight' for 70% of your day? This is the chemical cause of stress, now add to that the physical (breast implants, excess fat, misaligned spine, inflamed organs) and emotional (shame, fear, guilt, not enough, anger, grief) pieces and it starts to make sense…but it definitely doesn't make energy nor build health.

Methyl groups are needed to turn on the stress response but are also imperative to turning it off. These include things like Vitamin C, NAC, B Vitamins, magnesium, Zinc which you can get in food, but I also recommend you take it in high dose multi form as insurance, because food is so nutrient deplete today. When methyl groups are lacking, it creates a greater opportunity for toxins, inflammation, and other instigators to trigger bad genes. Toxic diets, lifestyles and various other stressors (whether chemical, physical, or emotional) can turn on bad genes by depleting methylation. On the

174

other hand, a healthy lifestyle, clean diet and natural environment can properly restore methylation and turn off a bad gene.

"Hence, your genetics are no longer your destiny."

Now do you see why earlier when I said, 'Just because you have the MTHFR gene doesn't mean your detox pathways have to suck'? is a myth? It's empowering to know you have it, but it doesn't mean you can't do anything about it, nor does it mean it's actually a gene that's 'acting dirty'. I'm double homozygous for MTHFR (got one mutation from both parents) and have the COMT, CBS, and more 'sucky genes', hence am a poster child for poor detox pathways, but because I support my body at the cellular level with this 5R protocol as well as the 5R gut protocol and emotional protocol, my detox levels are usually winning these days!

As you can see, the 5R's act as a guide to fixing the cell. But you can't stop here to achieve successful detox and restored health. Read on to understand the next component in the process of getting your life back.

Step 2: Opening and Supporting Detox Pathways

While continuing on with Step 1, you'll want to incorporate Step 2, which typically lasts three to four months and is just as important. Opening these downstream detox pathways includes strengthening the lymphatic system, kidneys, liver and gut before adding strong binders to the mix, as we do in in Step 3. What are these detox pathways?

Let me first start by saying I am fascinated by the lymphatic system. The body's ability to detox begins with *the collection of lymph nodes throughout our body, connected like highways,* which helps clear the blood of toxins and takes stress off the other detox pathways by pushing toxins further downstream for removal.

Did you know that Blood represents only 25% of your fluid volume and the other 75% is lymph? So why do we focus so much on blood testing when of all the body's 7 channels of elimination: the liver, lungs, colon, kidneys, blood, skin, and lymphatic system, the Lymph is the most critical? It acts as the master waste management of your body and does the heaviest lifting of toxins to be carried out, so you're not damaged by them.

Learning to love your lymph will help you not only prepare your body for detox pre and post explant to move out the combat signs of aging, reduce cellulite, radically improve your skin, release disease causing fat, boost your immune system, sense of vitality and more. These are the self-care secrets that have been practiced for thousands of years and are known to holistically heal the body, reduce the need for toxic anti-aging treatments and improve your overall appearance and outlook on life. Interestingly, the largest concentration of lymph tissue surrounds your gut, so it's critical to focus on healthy digestion to support lymphatic health and successful detox.

Infrared saunas and Full Spectrum Saunas are very powerful detox tools, and can open up the skin detox pathway, removing a lot of the toxic burden from the lymph. I go deeper into sauna protocols and specific sauna companies and types in the resources section of my website and my online programs. I also create custom sauna protocols for clients based on their labs, toxic load, mental/emotional state and medical history. Other great lymphatic detox ideas were discussed in the pre-explant section and include: rebounding, yoga, lymphatic drainage massage, deep breathing and high-quality supplementation.

The best thing you can do to cleanse your liver is to reduce the amount of stressors that congest it. Also, the liver can only fulfill *all* of its roles when we give the body what it needs to detox. There are two phases of cleansing the crap that makes us fat, fatigued, and frustrated:

- Phase 1 requires different foods and nutrients: more vegetables, plants, fiber, fruits, citrus, etc.
- Phase 2 requires more protein, amino acids, animal fat, etc.

If Phase 1 dislodges the toxins from their hiding places, and Phase 2 carries them out of the body, then a cleanse is not complete without arming the body with both sets of tools.

This is where juice cleansing falls short because there are very little, if any, fats and proteins included. The really cool part is that you can get an idea for how your body is functioning with both

177

of these phases, through two things: (1) by taking your neurotoxic score once a month to see how your body is improving (take the quiz on my website) and (2) genetic testing as well as exploring how your hormones, neurotransmitters and toxins are being cleared from your body, which I can see in the urine lab hormone tests I use in my practice. Unfortunately, your doctor won't know what this is, nor will it be covered by insurance. Reach out to me if you would like help with any of this.

Fourteen Foods that Cleanse the Liver

1. Garlic
2. Grapefruit
3. Beets and Carrots
4. Green Tea
5. Leafy Greens (DIM rich - estrogen flushers)
6. Avocados
7. Apples
8. Olive Oil
9. Alternative Grains (alternative grains like quinoa, millet, and buckwheat)
10. Cruciferous veggies – broccoli and cauliflower (also DIM-rich estrogen flushers)
11. Lemon and limes (citrus)
12. Walnuts (are omega 3's)
13. Cabbage

14. Turmeric (spices)

Step 3: Use Strong Binding Agents to Remove Toxins

This part of the process is least discussed in the world of cleanse fads. Welcome to the world of utilizing true binding agents. You may have never heard of binders before. Not because they're any less important, but because this is where most practitioners can really cause harm. Yet, this is the essential step that makes all the hard work come together. When I discovered zeolites that were tested properly and actually proven to work via tangible lab results, I was stoked. Unfortunately, the research I dug up on zeolites revealed that many brands and formulas were extremely toxic.

Most clinoptilolite or zeolite products that have been tested, test positive for heavy metal contamination. This is because zeolites are natural chelators in the environment and thus bind onto environmental heavy metals. You want to work with one that ensures the product is completely free of contamination.

As far as duration, I recommend to supplement with them for at least one year, maybe more-- depending on your toxic load, genetics and stress levels. Removing neurotoxins that have bio-accumulated in the brain over the years solves the mystery of why so many women suffer unexplainable symptoms, illnesses, have "tried everything" and still don't even feel well. It also resolves hormone imbalance, since toxic load is the root of it all, which you'll learn more about in the next Chapter on how to heal your gut and hormones.

Remove the interference and the body will do the healing: this is where true hope lies, not in man's manufactured chemicals.

Most practitioners don't help their clients achieve a cellular level of detox and rarely, if ever, get upstream to detox the brain. I see many clients who see specialists frequently, for treatments performed by high tech machines that claim to reset the brain yet have never been assessed nor treated for heavy metal and neurotoxicity. Yet, this is the root cause of illness (in combination with emotional trauma) and what it takes to allow the body to really heal. Remember, it is not the doctor, or even what you find in this book, but your body that does the healing: the healing comes from an innate intelligence, directed by the brain and nervous system. The cure is YOU. Any detox program short of clearing both toxins and trauma simultaneously will not last the test of time.

Furthermore, preventing re-tox, or autointoxication, throughout the entire detox process, is essential. Most of the toxins are transported from the cell to the liver and then dumped into the gut. Once in the gut, toxins must be transported out of the body so that they are not reabsorbed. Autointoxication causes dangerous symptoms most doctors will treat with medications and remains a common occurrence in most downstream detox programs-- another reason why using true binders during detox is critical to safely

180

getting results. Remember when I told you 90% of bile from the colon gets recirculated? If it doesn't leave, it gets reused and hence can re-tox you.

To summarize, your optimal health and vibrant self will only return once cellular functions are improved via the 5R's and if real detox agents (that actually have the ability to pull toxins from the cell) are used to avoid toxin redistribution. This is how many practitioners and clients get their lives back using the approach you are reading about in this book. The most advanced people have tried various type of cleanses, but they still aren't anywhere deep enough to actually fix and repair the cell, in order to truly get well.

Some of these 'downstream' cleanses include:

- A colon cleanse (good to help with constipation and clear toxins from the colon, but not heavy metal toxic load)
- A foot bath (good for edema in lower legs, but still not proven to effectively remove toxins)
- A raw juice fast or celery juice 'cleanse' (if using primarily greens without adding high amounts of fruit, you may achieve fasting benefits to support detox, at best)
- A coffee enema (good to move toxins from the liver and toxic bile complex, but not far enough upstream to pull toxins from the cells where they are stored)
- A bottle of chlorella tablets (not a true binder)
- Seven- to ten-day herbal cleanses (not true binders)

I did all of these and more, in over 25 countries, studying and mentoring under various type of Ayurvedic doctors, Chinese doctors, raw food leaders, Shamans, yogis, Craniosacral therapists and more over 8 years I was sick, until I got Breast Implant Illness. Thank God for this experience, because it was a huge influential wakeup call that really challenged me to go deeper in detox strategies and protocol, the silver lining in my suffering, because if I didn't get as sick as I did, I wouldn't have been motivated to go deeper and have the wisdom to help you get un-sick with the very best approach in the world.

Chapter 8: Heal – Trust Your Gut to Fix Your Hormones and Reclaim Your Power

You may have heard it said by Hippocrates, The Father of Medicine from over 2,000 years ago: "All disease begins in the gut" ... so it can end there too. But it's not enough to know, it's more important to know how and to actually do.

How many times have you been told you 'should' do something, but you don't? Part of it, is the more toxic your gut is, the less happy, motivating, peaceful chemicals you can make.

Eighty percent of your serotonin is made in the gut. This is your happy neurotransmitter. All disease begins in the gut. And harmonized hormones come from a healthy gut. If your gut isn't in good shape, how can it make happy chemicals for you?

Alongside the work you are doing to detox heavy metals from your body, you will also want to follow along with a balanced gut healing protocol, immune boosting regiment, and hormone optimization program which are conveniently all achieved in *one* place... The gut! Because let me tell you, breast implants do a number on your gut. In many cases, women report bloating that not much has worked to remedy.

Here's where our next 5R protocol begins:

R1 Remove toxins, bad bugs, viruses, heavy metals, radiation, bad bug waste and pathogenic triggers. Many cleanses just remove the waste from the waste, yet don't get deep enough to clear the source. Where they take residence varies in your body, therefore we want to ABC, *Always Be Cleansing*, so we can do deep drudging where many toxins have been stored for years, instead of just doing a simple one-off brush stroke. It can take six months to clear all phases of parasites, and two years to clear heavy metals so be sure not to stop after just one round. Detox is a lifestyle, not a transaction.

R2 Replace enzymes, HCL, bile support, digestive aids, etc. Supporting methylation with B vitamins supports the production of bile so your gallbladder can do its job as well. Especially if you are missing organs, (like your gallbladder) you should take a bile supplement, such as ox bile.

R3 Repair so as to not have to depend on digestive supplements and vitamins forever. It's *critical* that we regenerate the tissues that helps us absorb nutrients from food. Otherwise, you'll take fifteen pills for fifteen ills.

R4 Re-inoculate – I like to rotate probiotics for Candida busters and spore-based strains especially in the BII space, because we tend to need both...

R5 Rebalance – During the Rebalance phase, additional lifestyle choices are addressed, which affect the gut most. Sleep,

184

exercise and stress can all affect the gastrointestinal tract. Yoga nidra, healthy sleep hygiene, and being kind to yourself are key, in addition to a gut friendly diet.

There is definitely an art and level of mastery to this, which is why so many women are still sick years after explant—not to mention poor advice and misinformation, especially in regard to healing the gut.

Myth: I need to do a "candida cleanse" and/or "parasite cleanse" after explant to heal my gut.

Truth: Pathogens are there for a reason, usually due to poor immune function caused by toxins and trauma. Just killing bugs will not address the reason they are there (weak immune function, hormonal chaos, etc.). You must heal the root cause to heal the entire body holistically.

Parasites, candida/fungus, bacteria, viral load and everything in between are *most* common in women with breast implants.

Breast implants as foreign objects continuously activate the immune system, eventually resulting in immune dysregulation, as they overstimulate the system. Toxic chemicals and heavy metals in breast implants also trigger the suppression of a healthy immune system response. I often see depressed Secretory IgA on a stool analysis, which is the gut's main immunoglobulin and first line of defense in protecting the intestinal epithelium from endotoxins and pathogenic organisms. With depressed Sigma, the gut is left defenseless against pathogens, which results in the overgrowth of opportunistic organisms like bacteria, fungi, viruses, and parasites, as well as reactivation of once dormant pathogens such as Epstein-Barr or pathogens that cause Lyme disease. This causes further deterioration in virtually every system of the body.

It's not enough to simply go on a bug-killing spree. Many women have come to us having done this candida cleanse or that parasite purge and are no better off because of it. Not only do pathogens feed on heavy metals, but they actually serve the purpose of protecting you from even more heavy metal exposure by doing so. If the underlying heavy metal burden is not addressed, these infections will keep coming back over and over. By addressing toxicity alongside healing the gut lining and restoring immune function, we can successfully deal with infections, as well as consider the things that increase pathogenic overload to begin with.

However, Candida isn't bad per se, it's just bad when it grows disproportionately. Technically, we *all have* candida. The good news is that Candida Albicans is actually a helpful fungal yeast that resides in the mucus membranes of your mouth, intestines, and genitals. Its job is to assist with digestion and nutrient absorption and it lives harmoniously with a variety of other microorganisms in a healthy balanced body.

However, if the opportunity arises, candida can get big, gang up and can be a real troublemaker, especially in women with breast implants because of our high levels of toxic load

When an imbalance in your gut flora (also known as dysbiosis) occurs, it can cause candida to get out of control. Candida can multiply, poke its way through the mucosal barrier of the gut, and make its way into other areas of your body, causing all types of unpleasant symptoms.

In addition to breast implants, there are many other reasons why candida can over-populate in the body:

- Antibiotics – including prescription medication as well as those found in our food and water supply. Most water filtration systems lack the ability to detox these.
- Heavy Metals and environmental toxins
- A high stress lifestyle, adrenal fatigue, or poor sleep habits.
- Emotions (such as fear) on chronic overdrive.
- Cortisone and other anti-inflammatory drugs that compromise the intestinal flora.
- Birth control – 69% of birth control pill users develop candida
- Copper toxicity (coffee and birth control are big proponents of this)
- Estrogen dominance or high levels of estrogen in the body
- Higher levels of fat on the body.
- A diet high in refined carbohydrates and sugar

So, as you can see, conquering candida is more than simply getting rid of an infection, or treating a symptom, it involves a holistic approach to restoring balance and function to your entire body, the very principals that this whole book is based on. One of the most *invaluable* things I've learned through this training and clinical research is this: Candida is a symptom of an underlying imbalance in the body that, if left unaddressed, will grow back again, as a defensive mechanism to protect the body from more severe harm a deeper imbalance could cause.

Better said, candida grows... Because it *can* and *must*. As an example, I see *heavy* metals and excess estrogen backed up in the liver as the key drivers to Candida overgrowth. So, if these are not addressed, Candida will come back again and again... As will the symptoms it brings with it.

Parasites

There are various estimates of how many parasites we have in our body and what percent of us have them but suffice it to say that they are easily spread from animals and pets to human (please don't French kiss your dog or allow them to lick your face and body) as well as from human to human among various bodily fluids. They are everywhere all over our body not always because they are bad, but most often today because (like candida), they have to be. They're like the bottom- feeders mopping up the mess our breast implants caused, added to the toxic soup we live in today; from mercury fillings in our mouths, glyphosate in our foods and lead in our lipstick to aluminum in vaccines and copper in our birth control (oh and Silicone in IUDs), etc.

Parasites can range from microscopic amoeba to ten-foot long tapeworms. These parasites (and their eggs) can enter the circulation and travel to various organs, such as the liver, where they can cause abscesses and cirrhosis. They can also migrate to the lungs-- causing pneumonia-- and into the joints, brain, muscles, esophagus and skin where they cause hyper inflammatory processes.

Chronic parasitic infections are linked with intestinal permeability and leaky gut syndrome, irritable bowel syndrome, irregular bowel movements, malabsorption, gastritis, acid reflux, skin disorders, joint pain, seasonal allergies, food allergies and decreased immunity.

We can't just go on a parasite cleanse, without addressing heavy metal detox at the same time. The reason for this is because when metals are detoxed, parasites can be released. When you start detoxing metals, you start to strengthen your immune system and when your immune system works better, you can start killing off some of the parasites. One of the things I see commonly in women with BII, is a poorly functioning immune system in the form of Secretory IgA, which is the gold standard for fighting off infections in the gut. When that is low, infections are high, and toxins are high with it. So, supporting all three of those things simultaneously is key.

It is also important to reduce your exposure to these toxins and infections, as explained in Chapter 10. The toxicity of our environment supports the toxicity in the body, including accumulated heavy metals, parasites, biofilm, and molds. Many factors contribute to the toxicity overload.

Your "Anti-parasitic" Nutrition Plan

Parasites love *sugar* and everything that turns into sugar. So, the best way to starve the parasites is through using healthy fasting and cleansing strategies, while eliminating as much sugar and grains from the diet as possible. Obviously, for serious health conditions, it's best to work with a qualified healthcare professional who understands intestinal health issues.

Several herbs and foods act as very strong anti-parasitic agents. Extra virgin *coconut oil* is loaded with medium chain triglycerides that enhance the immune system in its battle against pathogens. However, I much prefer *pure* MCT oil because it's about 6 times more potent than regular coconut oil. Raw garlic and onions provide sulfur containing amino acids that are anti-parasitic.

Here are some other fun herbs that are powerful additions to your arsenal. Unique herbs and fermented beverages for a clean digestive system includes dried oregano and especially essential oil of oregano, which is extremely volatile and anti-parasitic. Use two to three drops of oregano oil in water with fresh squeezed lemon and drink it three times a day. Clove works just as well, so you could also substitute or use clove oil with oregano oil. Ginger, wormwood, black walnut are also commonly used in anti-parasitic strategies. Fasting with vegetable or *bone broth* and loads of garlic and onions is a great anti-parasitic strategy. It is also important to use fermented drinks such as fermented whey from grass-fed cows and fermented herbal botanicals such as ginger, oregano, garlic, beet kvass, kombucha, etc.

Other fermented beverages include coconut kefir and apple cider vinegar. These are powerful tools to help destroy parasites. They contain organic acids and enzymes that help to create an environment that is non-conducive to parasitic development.

Three things that can help deepen the detox for parasites:

- *Apple Cider Vinegar* – go to dianekazer.com/resources to get the recipe!

- *Coffee enemas* – yeeeehaw! The best way to get rid of the bad bugs that bring on immune system overdrive that paves the way for auto immune disease, allergies, bloating, frequent colds/flus/sinus infection/viral infections, etc., is to give them a fun ass slip N slide to show them the way out the door.

- *Colon-hydrotherapy* - There is a huge difference between these and enemas although they're both referred to as "colonics." An enema only reaches the rectum and lower part of the colon (sigmoid colon), whereas colon hydrotherapy cleanses the entire length of the colon, about 5.5 to 6 feet. Colon hydrotherapy is many times more effective than an enema. One colon irrigation is equivalent to thirty enemas. Whenever you do a serious flush like this, I recommend you do one session prior to and then one after, within a week or so. Or you can do one before, then enemas after, or the other way around. Just be sure you're keeping your colon walls extra open.

After the cleansing period, it is especially important to utilize high quality, fermented foods such as kimchi, sauerkraut and fermented veggies. These foods are rich sources of L-glutamine, an amino acid that helps rebuild the gut, and also contain very powerful strains of good bacteria, organic acids and enzymes that act like soldiers to defend your body from parasites. Continue on with bone broth as a source of nutrient dense macro and micronutrients, which parasites are also known to deplete. I recommend one eight-ounce cup of bone broth two times per day, as a method to rebuild the gut lining and enrich your body's ability to absorb and assimilate nutrients in the healthy foods you plan to consume at this time!

Parasites, candida, and bacterial overgrowth (like SIBO), all cause something called "leaky gut" which is super common today, in fact I would think it's next to impossible *not* to have.

What Is Leaky Gut?

Sad truth: It's estimated that 83% of Americans who have celiac disease are undiagnosed or misdiagnosed with other conditions. Six to ten years is the average time a person waits to be correctly diagnosed. And by then, they have likely amassed something called leaky gut.

Every auto immune disease is said to be rooted in a leaky gut, which it's nearly impossible to *not* suffer from, given the amount of chemicals and stress we are exposed to today. Hence to reverse disease and most common symptoms today, it's *critical* to repair this gut lining. The intestinal tract is like a fine screen or mesh, which only allows nutrients of a certain size through. The nutrients then pass into the hepatic portal blood vessels, which can bring nutrients to the liver, your chemical detoxification power plant.

In a leaky gut condition, the intestinal tract becomes inflamed and the selective permeability (letting only digested food particle through) breaks down. This allows the passage of not only normal digested nutrient building blocks (amino acids, fatty acids and simple sugars from carbohydrates), but also the passage of larger food particles, like larger chain proteins, fats, and carbohydrates, as well as toxins that were never meant to pass through. This can be likened to a window screen. If the screen is functioning properly with no holes in it, air will pass through, but

193

the flies, mosquitoes, and other bugs will not. In leaky gut, the intestinal barrier becomes inflamed. Instead of only letting the digested broken-down food particles through, the larger food particles and toxins enter, causing the immune system to become weakened and over stimulated. This is like the screen that now has tears, making larger holes that allow all types of insects to get through.

This presents a few problems. Larger chain proteins can trigger not only intestinal irritation and inflammation, but also all kinds of allergies, immune and autoimmune problems, and inflammatory joint conditions, like rheumatoid arthritis.

Leaky gut can also result in toxicity, since toxins leak through the "screen" of your intestinal wall (because of the larger holes produced by the inflammation). These toxins ultimately end up in the liver, your chemical detox plant. Unfortunately, your liver is then overburdened, and the toxins end up circulating throughout the body, causing havoc wherever they go. If the toxins deposit in the brain, you might have foggy thoughts, possible memory loss and/or confusion, and even the start of neurological disease like multiple sclerosis, Lupus, Hashimoto's, etc. If the toxins deposit in the joints, you will have arthritic-type pains. If the toxins deposit into organs that produce white blood cells (WBCs), your immune system will be weakened, making you more susceptible to illness, including cancer.

What Causes Leaky Gut?

1. Stress causes lack of blood flow into the organs, including the bowel, which can result in leaky gut.

2. Food allergy/sensitivity is probably the largest daily cause of leaky gut in America. Big allergens are dairy, animal products and wheat – anything you eat cooked day in and day out becomes an allergen. Bacteria *love* processed food, so ditch the pathogens, ditch the food cravings for good!

3. Parasites can be found in all of us, especially intestinal parasites. They come mainly from sushi, beef, chicken, fish and pork, but they are everywhere. Especially for you world travelers out there. While it's true that traveling to foreign countries is the easiest way to pick up these bad bugs, they are everywhere in our society today. Plus, we are living such a sterile, probiotic lacking life, the bad bugs win. Also, emotional stress depletes our immune system so it can't do its job to fight bad bugs off effectively.

4. Poor diet, usually manifested in eating food that is highly processed or preserved, or high in fat or sugar or animal content.

5. Toxic heavy metals – like metallic lead, mercury or cadmium – cause irritation to the intestinal lining. Especially breast implants that contain them.

6. Drugs have many side effects, 7-500 to be specific that can result in poor assimilation. Drugs kill the normal flora of bacterial growth in the bowel, allowing pathogenic bacteria to grow back in a greater proportion. Candida, or yeast, also overgrows in

the bowel, causing leaky gut. Other drug side-effects are corrosion to the gastrointestinal tract, causing the inflammation and leaky gut. Acne meds, birth control, skin meds and antibiotics are *very* yeast-inspiring, especially Accutane, which I took when I was eighteen. Talk about a train wreck!

7. Eating or drinking toxic food containing chemicals and/or toxins. When we eat or drink food containing chemicals or toxins this directly causes intestinal lining irritation and inflammation which leads to a leaky gut. This is primarily in animal products and dairy. More toxins as you eat up the food chain, at least sixteen times more.

8. Eating acid pH forming food causes stress on the digestive tract and on your total health. This includes cooked animal /dairy products, refined sugars, and flours.

9. Eating dead or deficient food causes very poor digestion because once you cook the food, the enzyme content of the food is destroyed This not only causes leaky gut but also greatly reduces one's total health. So, next garage sale … ditch the microwave ay? (and take enzymes with dead meals)

10. Gluten is like sandpaper to the lining of our small intestine. Talk about battery acid for our insides. How do you feel after you eat bread? Likely happy! But then *boom*, crash! Then you feel you need more. Addicted? You probably shouldn't be eating this junk.

In addition to all of this, I always recommend you use quality supplements to help heal the gut, here is a comprehensive list:

- Quality spore-based probiotic
- Mucosa building supplement with amino acids and dairy-free immunoglobulins, which also improve Secretory IgA immune levels
- Glutamine
- Collagen products
- Bone broth
- Betaine with HCL and digestive enzymes with food

There are *several* more advanced and customized approaches to take with clients depending on their pathogenic load, symptoms, heavy metals load, neurotoxic score and how long they had their breast implants, but for now this is the very baseline foundation to help heal a gut. A healthy gut also contributes to healing your hormones, since they are produced from a vibrant gut and high functioning, detoxed brain!

The other key is to avoid the things that contribute to leaky gut that I mentioned.

Speaking of hormones, how can we fix *these*? There's a common misconception that says, "If hormones are low, add hormones exogenously." But that's not a good idea in the beginning since, those suffering from BII are so gummed up with toxins, we may not even absorb them well and they could harm us or be expensive at best.

Heavy metals and toxic chemicals found in breast implants affect your hormones. Certain enzymes are needed in order to produce pregnenolone (the master hormone) from cholesterol, and then different enzymes are needed to convert pregnenolone down the line to make each of our steroid hormones. These enzyme functions are directly affected by certain metals and chemicals (many of which are found in breast implants and their shells). If your enzymes aren't working because of toxic exposure, you're not going to be making hormones! Additionally, some metals, like mercury, aluminum, and cadmium act as metallo-estrogens in the body. This means that they bind to estrogen receptors and mimic the effect of estrogen, causing estrogen-dominance symptoms. So, once you effectively detox the metals, your estrogen load should drop, and your other hormones will stabilize.

There is another major class of hormone disruptors which, when addressed, allow hormones to find their balance, again. These are called: xenoestrogens.

Resolving Estrogen Dominance

Prior to BII, I had been interviewed on this topic more than most anything else, because I believe it to be one of the biggest threats to our planet and our health. ED is affecting more Americans (and countries that follow USA trends) than ever in our history and it's evident when I test the majority of my clients. Unfortunately, these symptoms and conditions have become the norm:

- Painful, heavy, clotty and/or long periods
- PMS
- PMDD
- Mood swings
- Chronic fatigue
- PCOS
- Endometriosis
- Ovarian cysts
- Acne
- Weight fluctuation
- Menopause
- Migraines
- Breast cancer
- Hypothyroid
- Hair loss

I know what you are thinking "Hair loss? Isn't that a thyroid symptom?" Yes. And here's the connection. Estrogen dominance causes the liver to produce high levels of a protein called "thyroid binding globulin", which, as its name suggests, binds the thyroid hormone and decreases the amount of thyroid hormone that can be assimilated into and utilized by the cells. What does this lead to?

Low thyroid function and all of the negative side effects that come along with it...such as *hair loss*!

This is all preventable with the right labs, beauty routine, stress management, hormone balancing protocol and detox program.

Unfortunately, Western doctors are not trained to explore and address the root causes of ED, and in fact, most solutions they offer further contribute to it (like birth control, overuse of plastic, the SAD, HRT and more).

Check out the top ten ways we're exposed to synthetic estrogen and xenoestrogens (chemicals that mimic estrogen in the body):

- Water – Drinking and showering
- Plastics, even BPA-free kind
- Pesticides in commercial produce
- Dioxin – bleach used to make tampons white!
- Parabens – check your make up and personal care products.
- Phthalates – in fragrance and 'home' smell good items.
- Soy products
- Commercially raised meat and dairy
- Copper – Copper IUD's
- Birth control and hormone replacement

Birth Control and artificial hormones we're given to make us 'feel better' are short lived in two senses of the term. The relief is short lived and so too are we.

The number one cause of breast and ovarian cancer today is estrogen dominance from the myriad of synthetic chemicals we're exposed to today.

The Estrogen-Gallbladder Connection

If the liver is overwhelmed with too many other tasks (grossly common today), it can't properly and completely detox metabolites of estrogen, so they back up into the gallbladder and congest the bile ducts. With BII, the issue is compounded even further because breast implants are xenoestrogens. You may have had issues before and went to your doctor. The *worst*-case scenario is that you were told your gallbladder needs to be removed. In the meantime, your gallbladder may be trying to talk to you. It's using "words" like estrogen dominance, skin problems, acne, gallbladder infection, migraines, hot flashes, inability to break down fats, nausea upon consumption of fats, hormone imbalance, pain under right shoulder blade, inflammation under right rib cage ... If it's so bad that doctors are recommending surgery, I highly urge you to do your homework first. I've heard nightmare stories and hey, God gave you a gallbladder for a reason.

Contrary to what the doctors tell you, your health *will* be impacted without it. Not to mention, it's one of the most common emergency surgeries performed at ERs today...Without the ancillary advice to supplement with bile salts or other digestive aids to assist in emulsifying fats, which will be the newly acquired impairment.

Being that the majority of women today are on some kind of synthetic hormone or birth control, is it a surprise that the majority of GB removals are WOMEN? Not to mention, breast cancer. The excess estrogens back up into the next set of tissues neighboring the gallbladder and other detoxification organs that are also backed up. Yes, I mean the *lovely* lymph system.

"What the body cannot excrete, it stores, and *grows* into disease ... and *shows* on our waistlines, our skin, and in unpleasant symptoms around that time of the month."

This is one of the reasons I am such a big fan of castor oil packs, discussed in other chapters, to detox your gallbladder, reduce your estrogenic load and free up some toxins from the liver so your body can continue to release backed up toxins in the lymph as you progress through the cleanse phases. Allowing the gallbladder and liver to do their jobs, will allow critical pathways to open so that toxins will have a continuous exit strategy.

So how else can you remove xenoestrogens? By increasing your fiber load, especially leafy greens high in DIM like kale, collard, broccoli, cauliflower, Brussel sprouts. I recommend consulting with a practitioner on whether or not it's necessary to take a supplement with DIM or CDG, in addition to food. Often times the work you do with the advanced cleansing and gut repair in this book should be enough to release them – if done right, consistently, with the right formulas in the right order for a long enough period of time.

So how do I get more energy in the meantime, while also supporting my hormones?

Until then you can try adding some adaptogens to your daily routine. Add these to your shakes and smoothies, rather than take more pills. They help maintain a balancing or normalizing effect on your body, no matter what kind of stressor or agent is impacting you. Adaptogens also boost your body's resistance to stress and other environmental toxins and create equilibrium in your body safely and with no adverse side effects, even when used long-term.

Here are my *favorite* hormone adaptogen warriors, which are in many of my recipes in The Warrior Cleanse, such as my and many others favorite 'the Metabolic Mocha', as I believe it's easier to consume them in meals than supplement form:

1. Maca – if you're looking to get your mojo back, maca is the adaptogen for you! Used for thousands of years in the Andes, this ancient cruciferous root offers hormone balance, immune support, improved fertility, boosts your mood, increases energy, stamina, improves sexual function, memory and focus because it helps the body naturally adapt to those everyday stressors we've been facing.

2. Ashwagandha – Ashwa.... what? Ashwagandha! If you could restore your energy, look younger and reverse disease all in one pill, would you take it? Yeah, so would I! Enter, Ashwagandha. One of the most powerful ancient Ayurvedic herbs, Ashwagandha is often used to strengthen the immune system after illness, improve

thyroid function, treat adrenal fatigue (which we *absolutely* need after we laid out all of our stress above!), reduce anxiety and depression, increase stamina and endurance *and* stabilize blood sugar.

3. Reishi Mushrooms – I've been shroomin' with reishi for *years* now. Studies have repeatedly shown that reishi mushrooms have antioxidant abilities that strengthen the body's defenses against cancer, autoimmune diseases, heart disease, allergies and infections. Plus, reishi lowers the amount of toxins and heavy metals in the body, protects against viruses and lowers inflammation and chronic pain.

4. Cordyceps – This is probably my favorite after Maca and Ashwagandha. Prized for their natural ability to fight free radicals, infection and inflammation, Cordyceps are impressive disease fighting mushrooms that have been used for centuries to reduce symptoms of respiratory disorders, coughs, colds, liver damage and much more. They can even act like a natural cancer treatment in some cases, preventing the growth of tumors (especially in the lungs and on the skin).

5. Astragalus – With its roots in traditional Chinese medicine for thousands of years, Astragalus is a plant within the bean/legume family and has been known to boost your immune system, protect from both mental and physical stress, slow or prevent the growth of tumors and protect the cardiovascular system.

It is also a very powerful anti-inflammatory, containing antioxidants—plus it's great for anti-aging.

6. Licorice root – can increase energy and endurance as well as boost the immune system and protect the thymus from being damaged by cortisol.

7. Dong Quai – known as the "queen" of herbs for its amazing ability to balance women's hormones, Dong Quai is also effective as a blood replenishing tonic. It can be used by men to treat prostate health and for everyone, it creates energy, treats depression and is a great source of vitamins E, A, and B12.

8. Ginseng – is a potent adaptogen and is used to improve mental performance (bye, bye, brain fog) and your ability to withstand stress. It also has antioxidant and antidepressant effects and can help naturally lower blood pressure and blood sugar levels. Best part: it's an aphrodisiac!

9. Holy Basil – high up on the list of beneficial Ayurvedic herbs, Holy Basil, a.k.a Tulsi, naturally lowers elevated cortisol levels, helps regulate blood sugar and hormones.

10. Rhodiola – want to alleviate depression, stimulate the nervous system, boost mental alertness and eliminate fatigue? Rhodiola is your answer.

In addition to that, I am a huge fan of 'glandulars' for hormone support. I take both an adrenal and thyroid glandular which were game changers for me especially because as I was enduring my explant process, I also turned 40 so I was up against a lot.

I don't believe Hormone Replacement Therapy nor Bio Identical hormones are bad, I often find them unsuitable for the patient, as I mentioned before, most humans today, especially with BII, have clogged livers and toxic cells, so absorption is impaired, which means the hormones circulate around and land on other areas of the body, causing heart palpitations and growths of things such as tumors, cancers, fat cells, fibroids, etc.

Every case is different, so this is the Advanced level of support I only provide to one on one clients, as there is no such thing as blanket bio identicals. I will say I once was on thyroid medications, when I had Hashimoto's Hypothyroid, but I was able to get off of them and reduce my antibodies to the point of reversing my auto immune disease using the advice I am providing to you in this book!

Electric Magnetic Fields (EMFs)

Electric magnetic fields will increase your bad bug overload, if unaddressed. EMFs are invisible areas of energy, often referred to as radiation, that are associated with the use of electrical power and various forms of natural and man-made lighting. They are highest found in cell phones, computers, iPads, TV's, Wi-Fi, smart technology, our cars, microwaves, kitchen equipment etc. etc.

EMF amplifies the toxicity levels and impact of toxins released by bad bugs in our body by *hundreds* of times. EMF, plus mold for example, or plus heavy metal toxicity, or plus Lyme (all of which are increasingly common today) is the canary in the coal mine for many.

According to the research by Dr Dietrich Klinghardt "Wi-Fi increases the release of mycotoxins by 600 times." The more parasites you have, the more mycotoxins are released.

And in the BII space, I have seen higher levels of parasites because we have higher levels of heavy metals, so they are there to mop up the metal mess. In that sense, parasites are not bad, if they are there for this reason.

Mycotoxin is a Greek word meaning fungus or poison. The relationship between metals, molds and parasites is an if-then relationship.

These toxic wavelengths wire us literally, and alter our mood, how we process nutrients into the cell (mitochondrial damage), and hence alter our DNA. If we get to 5G, this will become eighty times worse, at least.

This relationship of heavy metals, parasites and EMF is a never-ending cycle of symptoms and suffering. Hence, we need to simultaneously go after all three at the *same* time. This is what sets our approach apart from everyone else. When you only address one or two of these without addressing them all, you won't get well, in fact you're likely to become even more un-well!

Here are my top five "easy to do, big impact" tips to reduce your exposure to EMF by about 80 percent:

1. Turn your phone on *airplane mode* before you fall asleep and be sure it's set to *off* mode for Wi-Fi and Bluetooth.

2. Do *not* hold your phone to your head when talking. Use wired earbuds and keep the phone at least one foot away from your body. Or use speakerphone.

3. Keep your computer one foot away from you too. Many studies are rolling out, revealing the research of how much EMF zaps us from laptops. If you need to use a laptop, consider an external keyboard and mouse, use it when not plugged in (it emits more EMF when it is), and *never* put it on your lap ... Ironic, laptop. Hm, your ovaries are *not* stoked on that. Infertility and tissue damage? No thanks.

4. Search outside of your home for a *smart meter*. If you have one, petition to remove/disengage it with your electricity company. It may cost you $5 more per month, but it's *worth it*. These machines have saved the utility companies from paying workers to visit our homes to manually read our meters, but at what cost? Our health!

5. Do an EMF emitting inventory, especially in your room. From TVs, iPads, computers, refrigerators, neighbor's Wi-Fi routers, etc. we are in *dirty electricity* central.

6.

Healing Is Not Linear

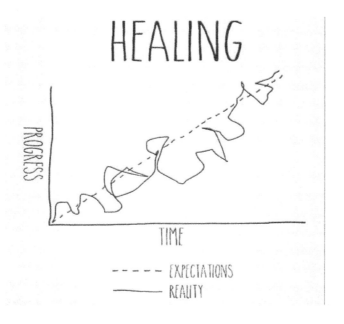

When skin issues arise, I invite you to see it differently. Especially with things that we women place heavy emphasis on, or what we feel defines our beauty: our skin, hair and nails. What is very common for women post explant through the detox process is: acne and skin issues.

This is absolutely something to *celebrate*. Here's why. This is your body's way of detoxing. And with some things, it gets a little worse before it gets better.

Here's the thing. The meds you've been on, the toxins you've harbored, the gut infections, the lifestyle you've been leading, and specifically the emotions you've suppressed your whole life, have finally been given permission to *leave* your body.

Why does acne need to be a *bad* thing? Or a reason to get discouraged? This is a fabulous sign your body is trying to protect you and talk to you. And this needed to happen for you to see so that you could see *this* differently. Remember, symptoms are self-love from the soul! So how are you talking to your body now that it's talking to *you*?

The number one ingredient in healing is patience.

Then when you think you have enough, give yourself more.

In addition, you can take more of the supplements with strong carbon binders, known to be effective at binding to toxins, such as the ones listed in the Cleanse Chapter.

The skin completely regenerates itself in four to six weeks and gut healing takes six months, at least. Ask yourself: Am I willing to be patient with myself under construction temporarily, in exchange for the chronic symptoms I would otherwise have permanently if I didn't fix them now?

I call this a *Hot Messterpiece*. You're allowed to be a Hot Mess and a Masterpiece at the same time.

When Can I go back to exercise?

This is a valid question I get a lot and the answer is it really depends on how quickly you heal as well as how toxic you were, etc. There really isn't a one woman answer here, but I will say, I highly advise you wait at least a month after your surgery, and above all, listen to your doctor and listen to your intuition.

Here's my story. 8 weeks after explant, I ruptured my Achilles tendon, playing soccer. I suspect it had something to do with the fact that I took Cipro the year before because I got sick while traveling though Peru for a month, and since natural treatments didn't work, I resorted to antibiotics, however it made things worse as most fluoroquinolones do. I highly recommend you avoid this class of drugs and ask for a different type of antibiotics or medication as an alternative, as they are known to cause major tissue damage, especially rupturing Achilles tendons specifically. You would say, I learned the hard way again! That's for a whole other book, so I'll keep it at that right now.

I'll leave you with this. When it happened, many of my Functional medicine doctors were also puzzled. 4 surgeries in one year? Because I had so many following my journey, and I wanted you all to learn from my ouchies, here's what I posted on what I learned in this process:

"I ended up having 2 surgeries on my Achilles. It was oozing the last 2.5 months since my first incision, resisting healing, so we were concerned about it

As we suspected, it was the stitches causing the infection. I took them home in my lil cup as a trophy. I'm so impressed at my defensive line for doing their job protecting me. BUT I'm a little nervous that my surgeon said couldn't remove the ones that were higher up and couldn't access so I am PRAYING my body doesn't react to those too. We were excited when he told us in the pre-op room "Your body obviously doesn't like artificial things, so I'm going to take them out, since you no longer need them" (we took that to mean he would remove them ALL, not just the ones my body mounted an infection around). They're made of Polypropylene (plastic) which may be what my immune system is rejecting, I suspect because my breast implants were made of similar chemicals.

Actually, the research I dug up when I searched 'Do breast implants contain Polypropylene?' here's what I found: "Polypropylene breast implants (or 'string implants') were only briefly available in the US before being removed from the market by the FDA in 2001. The thing about string implants that made them 'interesting' was that after implantation, the polypropylene would absorb water and its structure caused irritation within the pocket resulting in the body creating serum that continually fills the pocket."

...ok so if that's why they banned these implants, then why would they be using the same material for internal incisions? This material is the same as the Nalgene BPA free water bottles that does NOT dissolve?

I'm concerned my body will continue to 'fight' these stitches and further deplete my adrenals and immune system which per my last lab, were both hanging on a thread (my Secretory IgA and Cortisol stress hormones were extremely low).

I have little faith in the medical industry truly having our back on what is 'best' for our body. If we want to be healthy, it's now our job to become our own best doctor, by working with the right practitioners, asking the detailed questions and listening to our body."

So, I don't have answers for you here sisters. Just this: Be very, very mindful to ask questions to anyone putting anything in, on and around your body, then research what that could mean for you and your beautiful temple.

Chapter 9: Ignite - Free the Trauma, Find Your Voice

In this chapter, I will discuss the number one healing hack and 80% of the equation to reverse BII. By the time we get here, many of us have lost ourselves, literally and figuratively, along the way, and we are on a mission to discover:

- Who am I?
- What do I want to change about me and *how*?
- Why do I do what I do?
- How can I change what I don't like about what I do?

Everything we do is shaped by three things: *beliefs, values* and rules. We can speak mantras all day long. (Consciously). Yet, if we don't get to the weeds contaminating the roots of our tree (a.k.a. our foundation), it will be impossible to sustain the branches (acts of kindness, exercise, helping others, connecting, etc.). I created this module to help you connect to your subconscious mind, and what has shaped it, so you can be the observer of it, rather than the participant.

So, you can *literally* change your mind. How do we do that? Let's dive into it....

If you've been on a spiritual journey, you have likely heard this quote from Mahatma Gandhi:

"Your beliefs become your thoughts,

Your thoughts become your words,

Your words become your actions,

Your actions become your habits,

Your habits become your values,

Your values become your destiny."

Exercise: Take an hour or two to sit in nature on a blanket. Catch some fresh breaths. Maybe do some Nidra before you journal. Once your mind is clear and your body feels relaxed, press play on the audio, drop into these thoughts and note what comes up in your journal. Share with important people in your life such as your significant other, parents, kids, besties, siblings. Or, the big challenge, you share it with your *boss.* Oooh, *scary.* Unless you're your own boss, then even scarier LOL. Because, if integrity is a high priority value for you and you're not acting in this space behind the scenes of your own business, you realize you're self-inflicted sinning. Um...who's been there before? (Raises hand.)

As you write down examples of each, also ask the question and jot down:

1. Where did I learn this?
2. Do I like it?
3. Is this helping me?
4. Or hurting me?
5. Can I reframe/reword this?

#1 Beliefs

Beliefs are mantras and affirmations we say to ourselves all day. These have been inherited and embedded inside our subconscious, without realizing that they were mantras, way before we learned what a mantra is. They may sound like:

- I am
- I can
- I will

"I am" is a *happening now* statement. This is the real deal, the *championship game*, where you truly feel something or want to feel something and are acting as if is it is already happening, to call it into your life. The conscious brain will go searching for what the subconscious wants/resonates with and *voila* you are getting closer to manifesting that which you "feel" but maybe not yet "have" physically.

"I can," "I will" are *happening soon* statements. It's like "pre-gaming" yourself for the big game. It's your warm-up to the act of stepping into the "I am." Not as powerful but getting there. Oftentimes in this state, we tend to "blame" other things for our not being where we want to be ... And hear some *"If only's"* coming out. Perhaps inward, reflective of self, *or* outward. In other words, us not being where we want becomes either our own or other people's fault. Can you guess who gets the blame most? Those we pedestalize or have in the past – mom, dad, teacher, boss, relationship etc. They are also the ones who have the greatest potential to "hurt" us because we give them the power *to* hurt us by depending greatly on their approval, opinion and 'mattering' in their lives as a gage for our happiness. Depending on which continuum you fall on, you may not have the "outward blame" as much but, most often it's when this dies down in your mind, you know you are approaching the next level-- "I am."

"I should," "I need to," or "I 'have to" are all *happening never* statements. The are rooted in *shame.* It's crap. It's just crap. It's like saying "I'm trying" or "I'll try." To me, there isn't try, there's just do. It feels like shaming to challenge that concept but, in my experience when I have said it myself, it comes from a defended posture of shame itself-- shame for not just doing and accepting the process. It's still a "playing small" posture of "hiding from the I am," for fear that it won't work or perhaps we feel we don't deserve it. Typically, I see these as an "I'm not ready to work for it" statement. It's an "I'm comfortable in this snuggie right here in my comfort zone, and I just don't wanna." Real talk. I know it may hurt to hear ... But for real. These are powerless, codependent, and downright selfish.

Why?

Because as long as you are powerless, you lean heavily onto others to feel more power. Or to feed whatever insecurity you have to feel secure, whereas truly.... *You are the only person that can make yourself feel secure.* So which state are you in? The game, the blame, or the shame?

#2 Values

Values are like the "soul goal" foundations. Below is a list of core values commonly used by leadership institutes and programs. This list is not exhaustive, but it will give you an idea of some common core values (also called personal values). My recommendation is to select less than five core values to focus on – if everything is a core value, then nothing is really a priority.

Examples of Core Values:

Authenticity	Contribution
Achievement	Creativity
Adventure	Curiosity
Authority	Determination
Autonomy	Fairness
Balance	Faith
Beauty	Fame
Boldness	Friendships
Compassion	Fun
Challenge	Growth
Citizenship	Happiness
Community	Honesty
Competency	Humor

Influence	Recognition
Inner Harmony	Religion
Justice	Reputation
Kindness	Respect
Knowledge	Responsibility
Leadership	Security
Learning	Self-Respect
Love	Service
Loyalty	Spirituality
Meaningful Work	Stability
Openness	Success
Optimism	Status
Peace	Trustworthiness
Pleasure	Wealth
Poise	Wisdom
Popularity	

Integrity Reports

Use these core values to create your annual Integrity Reports. Writing these reports is a yearly ritual that forces you to think about how you are living out your core values in real life.

• For example, before I invite women to invest their time, money and energy in working with me, I examine what makes up who they are and what drives them. These are my core values I *prioritize and* look for in clients, knowing they would thrive working with me, therefore leading them to succeed in self leadership and self-healing. You possess values: coachable, committed, and conscious (above all to succeed)

- Have inner characteristics such as: curiosity, creativity and compassion (these are the 3 C's women who work with me in my CHI program dive deeper into igniting and sharpening to literally change their personal reality by reshaping their personality.

#3 Rules

There are so many interesting ways our brain creates restrictions around how we are 'allowed' to live our lives, based on our upbringing, and how we see the world which create these rules we live by to create order and structure. For example, here are some funny rules I learned/created:

- No showers unless you sweat.
- No relaxing until all the work is done and the house is neat.
- When a lot of info comes at you, it's OK to panic.
- When I get sick, I am more worthy of being loved.
- The world is out to get me, especially my mom (which I project onto women in my life when a situation resembles my mom).
- In order to "matter" I must work every hour of the day and if I don't I should feel guilty about myself.

- If I'm not helping people all the time, and saying no, I'm being selfish. Treat others like you want to be treated (golden rule).

These are all just ways of living and being we have either created ourselves or adopted from others and made them truths. Let's use this last one "the Golden Rule" as an opportunity for a rule reframe.

Reframe: Instead of treating someone as you would want to be treated, ask them what kind of support *they* need and treat them as they need to be treated so they feel empowered and strong enough to help *themselves.* I developed an acronym for this. When someone is struggling and asking for help, respond with, "I'm all E.A.R.S. to support you in this moment. In order for you to feel supported, what do you need most right now: 'Empathy, Advice, Reassurance or Space?"

- Empathy: "You're not alone," "I've been there too," "This is totally common," "You're going to live …" then you can share some of your "what helped" advice.

- Advice: "Here's what worked for me," "Maybe you can try too," or refer them to a professional or program to get help from experts. Be mindful that *most* people go straight to advice and skip the emotions and helping someone feel heard emotionally. This is a masculine trait and why many couples and friendships break apart because they feel the other person is trying to "fix" them when they just want to be "heard" which are the next two....

- Reassurance: "It's going to be ok. We'll get through this together. You've got a great family to support you. This is not the end of the world …" a.k.a. Sanity check. Reassurance that they're not crazy, etc.

- Space: Just listen to them. Be a body with presence, not trying to fix them, suggest anything or interrupt, just let them vent, cry, scream, whatever they need to diffuse their trapped traumas, hidden hurts, etc. Just don't let them throw it *at* you or PTF (point the finger) at you. That's when you'll need to draw some boundaries and let them cool off some and/or gather their thoughts.

How rules can hurt us?

- Finish your plate, there are starving kids in Africa (we overeat)

- I'll do something nice for you, if you do something nice for me (conditional love that keeps us disconnected from our hearts or from giving and receiving love because we're in a "that is my toy, in order to play with that you have to give me your toy first" tantrum).

- Always pretend like you know what you're doing (Imposter syndrome. Integrity breach. It takes a LOT of energy to wear a *ton* of masks to appear as though we're perfect and have our sh*t together)

Navigating the Ego to Free you from the Thoughts that Cause You Symptoms and Suffering

When you find yourself in a "should," "shame" or "sh*it" storm, this formula will show you how to get beyond the Primary emotion and into the secondary emotions, then the root thought or belief that is causing them.

Twelve Steps from Suffering to Sovereignty

1. What is the thought / statement?

2. Is it true?

3. How can I know it's true?

4. How do you react when you believe the thought? Identify the primary and secondary *emotions* (Ideally one primary and three secondary)

5. Where do you feel this emotion lives inside of your body? What *physical* symptoms do you feel from it?

6. What age does this emotion feel?

7. What memory is attached to this emotion? (where your ego said, "I'm never going to feel this again," that created a defended posture)

8. What memory beyond that do you recall being taught to believe a value, story, thought to be true and observed. Is it a learned behavior in response to others/self-opposing them?

9. What is your fundamental *need* not being met, causing this thought and ensuing emotion?

10. How is part of my ego benefitting from owning or believing this story (self-sabotage, martyrism)?

11. Who would you be without that thought?

12. What thought/belief/story can I replace this with?

This is called inner child, shadow, and ego work. Learning these core things about yourself can help you explore your deepest sense of shame, guilt and fear. This is the secret weapon to your source code and will hence help you to handle your inner self when parts of your trauma wounds show up, asking for healing.

You need to die before you can be reborn…and what I mean by that is…the parts of you that are attached to old stories, traumas, beliefs, what people, places, things represent to you need to die, so you can be free from the stories you make up about how they cause you to suffer. Only then can you rebirth a new you.

"You can't feel the height of your joy unless you've felt the lowest of your fears." Whatever you're not expressing you're suppressing and numbing out. To what degree does something reveal itself as an escape projected in the form of numbing devices? Food. People. Work. Alcohol. Drugs. Highs. And even healthy things like "bliss." Cleanse programs. Supplements. Exercise. Yoga. Sex.

Healthy or not, anything done in excess can be an escape if it's done from the intention of not feeling emotions other than what you've been socially taught is okay. Emotions which are: happy, fun, easy going, agreeable, successful ... whatever the F that looks like.

It's *all* about intent. What is your intention behind doing the things you chose to do?

Navigating all of this alone creates an endless loop of confusion because we can't see which key unlocks the prison door to free ourselves while we're inside. It takes mirrors and reflectors to reveal to us the power and gifts within, so we can see things from another perspective and gradually unlock the door that barricades us to our symptoms and suffering, sentenced to die slowly with our music still inside, unsung.

Do you want to die with your song still inside you? Gifts unshared? Messages unsent? Potential unrevealed? That is the true definition of living hell, would you agree? So how do we get out of this maze?

In my experience of coaching and being coached at the highest level in soccer, entrepreneurship, bodybuilding, personal growth, dismantling the ego, functional medicine, spiritual evolution and more, in order to detox the demons in our mind we must literally become a new person. We must shed aspects of our old self to create space for new and improved parts, yet often times that's scary AF to the parts that don't want to die. We resist change maybe because we're taught that we should fear it. That it's hard.

F*ck that! You know what's harder? Remaining the same and suffering through a life you're not happy with. And your ego may resist that now by saying "actually my life isn't that bad, I'll just remain the same, I should stop complaining, who am I to invest in myself? I have bills to pay, kids to feed. How selfish of me?" Until the next time you suffer the same symptoms and wonder if you'll either:

- learn to fully accept yourself as is or
- evolve and shift your reality by altering yourself, the person you are.

This is your personality which is crafted by the "I am" statements of who you *think* you are. Ninety percent of your thoughts are self-sabotaging and limiting, on repeat, like these:

- I am sad
- I am lost
- I am confused
- I am an idiot
- I am imperfect
- I am a fraud
- I am responsible for others' feelings
- I am only valuable when I help others
- I am not smart enough
- I am not pretty enough
- Or any I am *too* or I'm not (_____) enough...

Your cells a.k.a. prison *cells* hear that and biologically, chemically, physiologically react to all of it. This is 95% of your symptoms and suffering-- root cause right here (subconscious programming causing suffering). Not genes, not your parents, not the shitty food you ate ... Because all of that is chosen by and derived from your "I am*"* state.

When you shift those you shift everything, including *all* of the choices you make, which determine your results, which determine your emotional state.

But how?

"I've tried so many things, but I'm still not changed, so I'm highly skeptical that I even can." Take it from me. I am living proof! I took a "hit" financially, emotionally, mentally and physically so that I could teach others to free themselves from their fears with this new HIT formula.

HIT stands for Habituation with Intention equals Transformation

Sounds great in theory but how can you apply this from your same level of thinking that created the problems and prison to begin with? You must be willing to become a new person, practice it consistently, and have someone hold you accountable along the way.

The best way I have found to achieve what you want is to find a mentor, a person who is living life the way you want to live and study them. Model after them, become them, until you unbecome the you that is causing you pain, keeping you imprisoned. You must be willing to let parts die, which is a mourning process in and of itself and can be the main sticking point that prevents you from growth.

What is your relationship with death? Do you fear it? Do you fear dying? Your parents dying? Your pets? Your kids?

This is a fear within all of us and it will never be easy to lose things. However, forming a healthy relationship with death as do other cultures, such as India, will help you to let parts of you go, parts that are no longer serving you, so *you* can be in a "better place" as we all say when people pass on. Practice saying "those parts of me are in a better place" when you've released them? So how do you do that? It's scary to lose ourselves because we literally lose our mind and lose control and lose our center, which we've all been taught are loony bin worthy states to deprecate and medicate.

Nonsense!

Confusion precedes consciousness and grief precedes growth, so you *must* be brave enough to lose control and certainty by realizing you're not in control and to get comfortable with uncertainty. I call it falling in love with mystery and releasing the obsession of mastery!

Wanna know a secret? I was a f*cking *train-wreck* inside my head like most of the minutes of the day...no wonder I wanted to kill me. I was tormenting myself twenty-four seven. Love and approval were never an inside job for me. I got my needs met outside by others, a pattern shaped in my childhood. It wasn't my fault just like it's not your fault why you are who you are. I mean ... Kind of. We're fully programmed on how to think, feel and act by the time we are seven years old.

How you were treated as a kid is not your fault nor your responsibility. How you treat yourself now and others today is. So, to the bully parts within ... It's time to go!

INNERCISE: Inspired by one of my coaches, Mark VonMusser, king of mindset and self-mastery, it's time to look within at what you've already got going on!

Get a new journal and write 'Brag Book', on the inside of the cover. I want you to come up with and list 25 things that make you awesome, beautiful and perfect as you are. Feel what comes up for you as you are doing this. Are you celebrating what you're writing? Judging it? Hearing that 'Who do you think you are?' voice? Who's voice is that? When I first did this, I tracked it back to my mother, as do most of my clients.

What the literal brain will do is lump celebrations in with bragging, and prevent you from ever doing it again, because you'll do anything to prevent that inner b*tch judge voice that just wants to keep you small. This is just a little taste of 'shadow work' where you get to experience the moments you put yourself in the shadow of parent or caregiver, deflecting your greatest gifts, so they didn't have to feel bad about themselves, while you celebrated you. 'How dare they be happy, when I am sad, simmer your excitement down', is the message our inner child hears. And so it goes, we walk into adulthood, as giant a$$ holes to ourselves, struggling to celebrate our gifts or feel grateful for others. Gratitude is the greatest cock blocker (or should I say titty blocker) of fear. You want to cultivate courage? Get grateful for your strengths, the beauty you already maintain and the gifts you came here to share with the world?

How to Let Go and Let Die

I can absolutely say to my former passive aggressive, excessively codependent, Princess, needy parts that I had *many* conversations down this path from fear to freedom.

They were unwelcome tenants for many years and along the way, no matter how much they missed rent, flooded the house (inflammation), broke doors (digestive valves open), put holes in the wall (leaky gut) and kept the neighbors up fighting (insomnia)... I let them stay because I thought "Well, they are a part of me and I should love who I am, right?"

Not if they're disrespecting you!

So little by little I stood up to these "toxic tenants," first by sitting down and slowing down enough to be present with them. Some tenants were sad. Some were lonely. Some felt abandoned. Some were really f*cking angry. All micro fragments of my inner children to my current macro self were playing out old tapes through the lens of unresolved emotions and trauma.

It took time to talk to each one of them differently and uniquely, so they felt heard. And once I did, they calmed down. They stopped acting out. They saw things differently. They upgraded their lens from chaos to clarity.

They shifted their energy to being more helpful than harmful. Constructive not destructive.

Loving versus loathing.

And in order to make this shift, their perspectives had to *die*. Not their whole identities.

They just needed to be heard to be healed. And now... I am teaching this to others.

Through the maze of my suicidal thoughts, alcohol addiction, DUIs, co-dependence, excess, overachieving, workaholism, and perfectionism, I discovered my light by meandering the sharp edges of my darkness. I learned that running from your fears consumes you. It steals your joy, depletes your hormones and cock blocks your connection to your heart and others. We spend so much time and expend so much energy running from our fears that we claim to not have enough energy left to run for fitness, or metaphorically, run toward our dreams and a life we want!

Fun ponder: What if every time you ran during a workout you imagined you were running toward something, an intention you would realize at the end of your path? Running for purpose and with intention! I'm going to develop a treadmill where you plug in the dream instead of the distance.

I hope this is making sense. Is it resonating? Do you feel it in your body rather than over analyzing it in your mind? This is *key*. Nothing changes if you're simply "thinking" about it. That's what created the problem: in yoga we call that Chitta vritti – monkey mind. It will always make you dizzy if you live here. Once you bypass the mind and get into 'selves' within you by purifying the filter through which they see the world, you will improve the cells that shape you and literally shift and upgrade your entire health and vitality. This is where disease and handicaps miraculously disappear. In other words, you must feel it to heal it.

So how do you do this?

First off, I do not recommend you go about this alone.

It is *vital* to surround yourself with people who reflect the good within you because they have discovered their own. Their presence will resurrect the dormant love trapped beyond your fears that you can one by one let go of, through experiential moments reminding you that your past can die so your dreams don't. Is this codependence? No, it's interdependence! It is a *literal* human need to be connected to one another! This is okay, okay?

- Have coaches that have weathered the booby traps and can guide you down the path of safety, so you don't have to fall into them yourself. And there are many. As time presses on and the wolves in sheep clothing, rooted in greed, increase by the day, understand that there will be more. Yet, it will be more difficult to avoid fakes, falling, failures and financial setbacks without guide warriors who have won their own war and are ready to masterfully assist you to win your own.

- Try on love for size. Give relationships or partnerships a go! Allow me to be specific. I'm not talking about toxic people who numb out, avoid growth, lean heavily into religion and rigid rules, judgment or PTF. I'm referring to unionizing intimately with another who reveals unhealed aspects within you. Someone you can get complete with and transcend alongside, within the container of a relationship

- Having both a mentor and a lover is your superpower for growth, freedom, and joy! I myself don't date or engage in relationships with anyone unless they have or are open to engaging the support of an experienced coach. Because merging relationships as coach and/or parent *do not* work. If you want a healthy relationship, that is! If you parent and coddle him like a mother, he'll sleep with other women because he doesn't want to be a mofo (bad joke). Today more than ever, with all of the rejection fatigue, and temptation, it takes courage and patience with *yourself* to be in a loving, evolving relationship, because you must set aside your fears from the past and do it anyway, believing that this time it will be different because *you* are different and you're attract from a different and deeper more divine, balanced state within yourself!

Until you embark on these two ships – mentorship and relationship, you'll be a lost ship at sea, blind to the winds, in a fog, riding endless waves never knowing where land is, so you can one day get grounded there. You'll never know the true depth of the toxic tenants that live within you nor the greatness or gifts that are yearning to shine!

And one day after you've boarded these ships and taken many journeys around your inner world, you'll learn to let others steer their own ships and will be confident and experienced enough to steer your own ship, toward calmer sees, joyful and *free*!

Healing Past Trauma

The women we have treated who have the constellation of symptoms known as Breast Implant Illness, share a common thread of trauma. They place a *lot* of emphasis on what other people think, others' judgments about them, and fitting a certain mold of what they think they need to be to be loved, respected and accepted. These are deep pain wounds that have shaped stories and thoughts that impact choices, originating from:

- Ego-based fears
- Trapped emotional traumas
- Spiritual stuckness
- Heart blocks
- Pleasing other people

- Crazy busy lives
- Over-giving
- A sense of lack in life
- Misalignment with occupation and purpose

The emotional trauma leads to the physical trauma which is in this case installing the breast implants and the cycle continues since the energetic signature of trauma was never properly resolved. What I have seen is that once we are able to support women post explant and on the other side of BII, they find peace within themselves, forgive themselves for their past (toxic) decisions and finally are free from the torment that they are not "doing," "looking" and "acting" enough ... Because the trauma has been released from their physical body and energetic field ... Not to mention the physical trauma of having surgery, which is equivalent to being attacked by a bear.

Confronting Our Shame

This chapter is more so for women who get breast implants for enhancements, although also for women who would be mortified at the thought of not having breasts post mastectomy, especially after considering all of the new research on what implants are doing to women's bodies.

When I first got into connecting into the energetics and psyche of women who had breast implants, they were surprised at what I discovered. The majority of women were disconnected to the root of *why* they were incentivized to get breast implants in the first place. They thought they "just wanted to fit in their clothes better" or "even out their lopsided breasts" or "lift their saggy socks" which in their words was omission of shame, which is defined by Brené Brown as:

"...The intensely painful feeling or experience of believing that we are flawed and therefore unworthy of love and belonging – something we've experienced, done, or failed to do makes us unworthy of connection."

Shame equals flawed equals "I need to fix something about my body."

According to a study conducted by Dove Cosmetics, 96% of women don't think they are beautiful. And it's no wonder. Most magazines spend two hours photoshopping *one* image. So, this is an epidemic. We are programmed for perfection, and anything less than, we are culturally conditioned to "fix it."

In a nutshell, the desire to be "perfect" is the ego's breeding ground for shame, which we have become addicted to as an identification (a false one) of who we are ... Or rather who we "think" we are. Society has shaped us as such, so when we don't do it perfectly, we give ourselves permission to shame ourselves, fueling the ego's desire to be right. Then our brain responds accordingly with stress hormones and neurotransmitters like dopamine, which our physical body literally becomes familiar with, and eventually addicted to. The vicious cycle of perfectionism, and the plastic prison we are all in. Wanting to stand out and in doing so, fit in at the same time. How confusing. Help maintain a balancing or normalizing effect on your body, no matter what kind of stressor or agent is impacting you. Boost your body's resistance to stress and other environmental toxins. Create equilibrium in your body safely.

It starts with the "not enough" narrative from our upbringing, which morphs into the "bigger boobs" brainwashing and the "toxic treatment treadmill" to keep up with the women around us that are anti-aging obsessed, yet mentally depressed and financially repressed.

It's not our fault. This is *years*, centuries, of ancestral shame being passed down through generations of women. According to work of neuroscience imagineer, Dr Joe Dispenza, this inherited shame is more potent at influencing disease and toxic body dysmorphic based choices (like breast enhancements/implants) than genetics.

Did you know that the thoughts you have today are 95% the same as the thoughts you had yesterday? In other words, 95% of who we are is a set of automatic subconscious patterns. 95% of everything you think, feel, and do is controlled by the "programs" that run in your subconscious mind. 90 to 95% of who we are by the time we're thirty-five years old sits in this subconscious memory system in which most of our habits and behaviors exist.

So, where did we learn these patterns? How was this subconscious mind shaped?

237

By our peers, partners... But *mostly* by our parents or caregivers, those who were most responsible for raising and parenting us. Our most influential role models had the most impact until age seven, which is when our internal hard drive has been mostly engineered.

Most of this subconscious programming was shaped in the first seven years of our life. From the last trimester of pregnancy to age seven, we exist mostly in theta brain wave space (a.k.a. hypnosis), which is the most receptive space for our subconscious mind. We are essentially sponges.

So, think, *really* think for a moment, what you were exposed to as a child? What did you watch on TV? Read in magazines? Cereal boxes? Play with as toys? Wanted to be for Halloween? These are all the icons we are programmed to idolize and want to become when we grow into adults. And if we don't, we feel imperfect, a sense of shame for not being who we were hypnotized into believing we should be in order to feel accepted, adored, and approved of by others.

Shame if we're not shaped like Barbie, perky-breasted like Pamela Anderson, wrinkle-free faced like Hanna Montana. Or even slightly enhanced like our girlfriends who just wanted a little makeover. This commonplace perception that we are in constant need of alterations is what I refer to as the "Perfection Parasite" that sucks the life out of us, consumes our joy and threatens our evolution.

The fear of not looking perfect, or doing things perfectly, or 100% is the single reason most will hide in shame or never take first steps toward positive change... Which is more of a failure than trying, falling, getting up, learning, discovering, and trying again!

So then, we either suffer in silence, in shame ... Or we spend tens of thousands of dollars on expensive cosmetic surgery to "enhance" our look because the studies show that "over 90% of women reported greater confidence in their body after they got breast implants."

What the studies *don't* tell us is this: Breast implants all bleed, eventually make us sick somehow, causing symptoms of varying degrees, depending on the woman and hence, cause them to experience an even deeper sense of shame, in the form of self-betrayal. We may feel upset with ourselves for ever thinking we needed to cut ourselves open, to appease others, because we were programmed to believe we weren't (beautiful) enough.

I will leave you to journal this exercise:

• What conditions need to be present such that you would be enough?

• What does enough look like?

• What does enough feel like?

• Does the voice of approval come from within or from others?

• Where did you learn the definition of beauty?

• What would you rather beautiful look and feel like?

- What would it take for you to release your previous definition of beauty and replace it with this new one, to finally free yourself from the beauty bully within?

- What would you be able to accomplish if your beauty bully within were no longer beating you up from the inside out?

- What am I willing to let go of to birth this new life into reality?

AND...

- What do breasts represent to me?

- What do breast implants and having large breasts afford me?

- Who am I without my breast implants?

- What will I lose?

- What will I gain?

- What am I afraid of?

- What am I excited about?

- What story or belief do I want to release on the day of my surgery?

These exercises will tell you a lot about yourself, your why, and who you think you are, as well as where your judgements came from, which is to say, where you first gave your power away.

This is just a start on the surface to scratch the itch to challenge your "inner bitch", and is one of my favorite, as well as most effective ways I help women in our sessions to free themselves from the plastic prison they have been in for a very long time!

I challenge you to share this with the world, if you dare. I would love it if you tagged me as well. This is how we change the world, by sharing from our hearts, revealing our darkest fears. This is when you crack open to let love in, and feel what life is really about. By shining your light, you will motivate other women to do the same!

Chapter 10: Advanced Detox, and Continuing beyond Your BII Journey

In this chapter, you will find a tremendous amount of helpful information for options to deepen and improve your pre-explant journey or post-explant recovery.

There are guides to help you customize your experience.

Take notes, talk to your doctor, reach out to me ... I are here for you. Speak up so I can help you continue to customize it deeper each time, as it's impossible to nail down immediately, considering all of the moving parts inside of your body as it interacts with your environment, thoughts and lifestyle. This is one reason I like working with women prior to explant, because I know their body well and am familiar with how it reacts, their mind, labs, etc. so I can better support them with these details when the time comes.

Here are some of the most common questions I use to help clients unearth and customize on the journey to explant and beyond.

When to Start Sauna Post-Explant?

It's a good idea to wait one-month post explant to start sauna use. It takes a lot of energy to both heal from surgery and detox the body, so we don't want to take energy away from either of those things. This assumes you don't have any complications post-op such as difficulty with wound healing, infection, hematoma, etc.

See more info below on my favorite strategies to maximize your detox experience in the sauna.

Rebounding – How Soon after Explant?

Please consult your surgeon for a recommendation on when you can start rebounding. Light exercise is fine at one month, but since rebounding puts additional stress on the incision site, it's best to consult with your surgeon on this one.

Lymph Drainage

You can start lymph massage and/or dry brushing right away after surgery, avoiding the incisions and breasts for the first month. Moving the lymph can help keep toxins and nutrients moving through the body. Your lymph doesn't move unless either you're moving your body (such as with rebounding) or you move it manually. If you're stagnant, your lymph will be stagnant and that can mean toxic build up in the lymphatic tissue. Keep it moving!

Intravenous Nutrition: Does It Work for Post Explant?

IV vitamin C and glutathione have been shown to be very beneficial after explant (and possibly even before if your surgeon okays it) for preparing your body for surgery, tissue healing, immune and adrenal support after surgery. Always consult your surgeon first.

HBOT and How, When, How Often to Use?

HBOT stands for Hyperbaric Oxygen Therapy. It increases the amount of oxygen your blood can carry and has been shown to be very helpful for tissue healing, fighting infection, pain management, and establishing a blood supply for a fat graft post-op. There are also benefits to using it pre-op as well. The possible investment for that would look like this: $100 per session (one thousand dollars for a ten-session package). If time and money are issues, you can do three times per week for two or four weeks after surgery, which is what I did.

Because the benefits of HBOT are systemic and it has been used to treat a vast array of conditions, if you cannot afford it immediately after, there still may be great benefit to you down the road as well. Insurance does not currently cover this for post explant. You will find a video I made on this in my Resources section.

Oral Infections

It is said that over 70% of disease today starts in the mouth. That's why it's *that* important. But when should you address cavitation, root canals and implants post explant? Breast implants are just one source of toxicity. We need to address them all. That being said, I think it's important to give your body a chance to heal and recover from surgery before thinking about addressing other sources of infection or toxicity that are still an issue. So, I recommend you find a biological dentist (important) who can help create a plan for you regarding cavitations, root canals, dental implants (if they're a problem), and address them correctly and safely. If you've ever had a root canal or tooth pulled, there is a chance you could have a cavitation, which can cause systemic chronic illness. Amalgams are 50% mercury and off-gas into the body around the clock

They both need to be addressed if present. My thought is to wait about three months post-explant before having another stressful procedure. You'll be better supported and prepared for this by implementing the detox I discuss in this book prior to addressing these types of stressors. You can find a biological dentist on the website: http://iaomt.com/ Keep in mind, these are far more expensive than regular dentists and usually don't take insurance. When I work with clients, I have excellent sources of practitioners that have saved them $10,000 + on similar treatments than premium doctors charge, so use your discernment, shop around or you can always contact me, and we can discuss customizing this for you and shopping around. It's challenging to know what to look for, so I want you to feel safe in reaching out to me, knowing I have done a lot of homework here, so can navigate you around the potholes toward the pot of gold heehee!

Silicone Detox

If you have breast implants, you can bet that you have silicone in your body, yes even if you had saline implants, because remember the outside layer is silicone. We can detox this using the supplements I have listed out for you in my Resources section. There are currently no reliable labs available, nor do I believe it would provide any value. It wouldn't change the detox plan I recommend to you. Why? In functional medicine, there are some safe scientific assumptions we can make, and oftentimes lab testing can be inaccurate and misleading. I treat the client, her symptoms, her medical history and her goals, period. The treatment protocol should not be exclusively based on lab results, which is unfortunately what most doctors do today, to the detriment of the patient (you). This is why you dread the 'Your labs are normal, we don't know what's wrong, it's all in your head, take this toxic prescription to band aid your symptoms, so you don't feel what you're creating with your psychosomatic thoughts'

Bonus to Watch: on the truth of the Medical Device (and Implants) industry. Powerful Documentary *the Bleeding Edge*.

My 9 Step Sauna Protocol

In a way, the skin is like a third kidney, in that toxins can be eliminated in the sweat, similar to how they can be eliminated through the urine. Far-infrared saunas are the most effective for sweating. Saunas are also a simple, fairly inexpensive, and enjoyable way to detox. Here are a few important strategies for getting the most out of using a sauna.

1. *Increase your circulation before getting in a sauna*: It is best to do something that increases circulation. If tolerated, you can use a rebounder, a treadmill, or other means of exercise to increase circulation. You can also take niacin thirty minutes before to flush the skin. You may need to start with a small dose of niacin at first and increase as tolerated.

2. *Ease into it*: Because you are toxic from breast implants, you'll want to start off slow. If you are new to infrared sauna use, I recommend starting off with every three days for three to four weeks and gradually increasing from there. Sessions three to five times per week is optimal to work up to. You can see just how toxic you really are by taking the Neurotoxic Questionnaire. The higher your score, the more toxic you are.

3. *Set time limits*: The amount of time spent in a sauna detox session may vary depending upon your tolerance. To get your body accustomed to infrared therapy, start with fifteen-minute sessions every three days. Gradually increase toward forty-minute daily sessions in the optimal temperature range. You can stay in for up to an hour if tolerated, but I don't recommend sessions longer than that. Listen to your body. Be aware of excessive detoxifying. If you begin to feel symptoms such as nausea, fatigue, or flu-like symptoms during your sauna session, get out and hydrate with sole

water. A general rule is that if you feel worse after a sauna session, then it was too long.

4. *Hydrate each day* you are planning to use your sauna. Make sure your water intake increases. The sweat produced in infrared saunas is 80 – 85% water, so it is important that before, during, and after your sauna detox session, you drink plenty of water to rehydrate. As a general guideline, I recommend drinking at least half your body weight in ounces per day. On days you use the sauna, increase that by eight ounces before and eight ounces after.

5. *Replace minerals lost:* You're also losing minerals when you sweat, so it's important to replace them! I like to make sole water and add half a teaspoon to my water before and after sauna use. One really important mineral that can be depleted is magnesium. Everyone with chronic fatigue, heavy metal toxicity, autoimmune issues, or any chronic health issue is going to already be deficient in magnesium. I recommend supplementing with magnesium, 400-800mg per day.

6. *Use an intestinal binder:* Many people are unaware that only 70% of the detoxification effect of using an infrared sauna is from sweating. Researchers have found that 30% of detoxification happens internally due the effect of the infrared rays' resonant frequencies penetrating the tissues. This causes the cells to detoxify, and the toxins are then processed through the organs of elimination and out through the stool and urine. Taking intestinal toxin binders

before sauna use is absolutely necessary to absorb the internally mobilized toxins. See the Resources section for the binders I like.

7. *Include Sauna as part of your detox program, not as a stand-alone option*: Heavy metal detox is so often done wrong. There is a proper way to go about this and when done correctly, it really works. Some doctors prescribe IV chelation to remove heavy metals, which puts a true chelator in the body and removes a lot of metal at once. It works, but the problem is that it causes a lot of redistribution of metal back into the brain and other places. *Not good.* IV chelation can cause people a lot of harm. Alternative medicine doctors are using things like cilantro and chlorella (called the metal-magnet), which really do nothing. I'm not against cilantro or chlorella as superfoods, but they are *not* metal magnets. They won't pull the metals out of your brain, either. There are also herbal products practitioners are using that are only weak chelators at best and cause more redistribution of metals. That's what I call the "leaf blower", causing metals to move around the body, but not actually get out of the body. **Bioaccumulation of heavy metals in the brain is one of the main reasons people get sick from breast implants and they don't know it, because for many women it takes years for them to get sick.** One day the bottom falls out, which I call the perfect storm. There *is* a way out and removing the source (breast implants) is part of it but detoxing afterward is equally important. Infrared sauna should be part of a detox program, but not the only thing you do. You should be supporting your body's detoxification

organs and using true binders that can actually cross the gut lining and cell membranes to gently chelate toxins in the body and brain, at the cellular level. Full Spectrum or infrared saunas can be a great adjuvant to this kind of detox program.

8. *Find a comfortable temperature*: Preheat the sauna and begin a session when your sauna reaches 100°F. The optimal sauna experience occurs between 100° and 130°F. The level of heat isn't as important as the sweat. Whatever temperature you develop a good sweat at is the right temperature for you. For some it will be 100 and for others it will be 130+. Many chronically-ill individuals have a hard time tolerating heat or are unable to sweat, especially early on. Because 30% of the detoxification from sauna use happens internally without sweating, using a sauna at a lower heat setting without sweating is still effective. Even if you are only able to tolerate sitting in a sauna for a few minutes, it can still be helpful. Over time, most people are able to build tolerance to higher heat and length of time. For those who are unable to sweat, this can also improve with gradually increased use.

9. *Rinse off immediately*: After each sauna detoxification session, dry off with a towel. It is best to cleanse the body with soap in a hot shower to prevent re-absorption of the toxic sweat. You can finish the shower with cold water to close the pores. I like to get to the shower as quickly as possible after a sauna session.

Chapter 11 - Detox'ing Your Home, Cleaning, Beauty & Personal Care Products

*"Since 2009, 595 cosmetics manufacturers have reported using 88 chemicals that have been linked to cancer, birth defects or reproductive harm in more than 73,000 products." -**California Department of Public Health***

By now you know that it's not just about the toxic silicone and plastics in breast implants causing you harm. What you consume-- whether food, drink, skincare, the air you breathe, your home environment or any personal care, it's important to know that you are most likely exposing yourself to unwanted toxicity. Unfortunately, since World War II, new chemicals have been introduced every year and it's fair to estimate they're affecting every bit of your health and recovery. What's just as scary is that cosmetics and other personal care products are some of the most unregulated by the US government. Even with FDA recommendations, compliance is completely voluntary and rarely even monitored. So, in a (plastic-free-packaging) nutshell, it's high time for you to get promoted to Defensive Captain-- of your very own anatomy. Now, it's your new mission to become aware of what you're putting *in* your body and *on* your body!

You may have heard highly-processed food be referred to as "Franken-food"— maybe you've even heard me use that term in one of my videos… It's admittedly not a great image… Those beefed up flavorless conventional tomatoes might as well have wires hanging out of them. Now I want you to add "Franken-beauty" to your lexicon of imagery. Everything we inhale or apply to our skin also gets absorbed into our bodies— into the bloodstream and fragile microbiome-- forcing our liver into overdrive to expel said toxins. These conventional personal care products can cause a whole host of side effects, from hormone disruption and allergies to reproductive harm and even cancer. What's worse is, overtime, they bio accumulate-- so it's essential to ditch them as fast as you would an abusive boyfriend!

Some women complain about tossing their favorite drugstore beauty products. Over and over, they say, "but this conditioner works just fine, it leaves my hair silky smooth. And it's cheap!" Or "This moisturizer plumps up my skin and makes it feel softer." However, the industry manufactures these products in such a way that makes them appear to be working, when in reality, they aren't. The chemicals help to coat your skin or hair shaft, building a polymer layer which provides the illusion of smoothness. What about "sulfate-free" or "phthalate-free" labeling? Don't be fooled by luxury items or "green-wash" marketing tactics. No matter how pricy or inexpensive, brands will utilize harmful ingredients for the sake of shelf life and the deception of efficacy. Some may even contain habit-forming compounds, leading customers to continue shelling out the big bucks, allowing a free-flow of loyalty purchases for many years to come. Not anymore!

About 80% of personal care products aren't even tested for human safety. This isn't about being perfect and fear mongering yourself to the point of obsession. I (and many women I work with) literally became beauty toxin Nazis when we first learned about this. It's tough! While you don't want to subject yourself nor your loved ones, what WILL happen is this: you'll start to see them everywhere-- in public places, gyms, airports, grocery stores, etc. People will likely buy gifts for you that you'll never use. You'll hop into someone's car that has a Glade plugin or some other artificial scent that might restrict your respiratory tract and olfactory glands, causing itching, sore throat and headache.

This happened to me once when I was double whammied on a business trip to Arizona, where I rented an AirBnB and commuted to the conference center every day. After the third night, I awoke to a huge headache and was led to wonder why. I hadn't deviated from my healthy routine. My intuitive sense got me curious about what fragrances and cleaning irritants might be lurking in the home, so I went on a hunt. To my suspicions, I discovered hidden fragrances in every room, with artificial sticks and Glade plugins. Combine that with most every car hire's artificial scent product plugged into their vents. I'm so sensitive to fragrances, it's like an insta-headache for me.

So, how do you get away from all of this?

Let's begin to examine the myriad of toxic ingredients pervading our convenience store aisles and department stores. Particularly, as they pertain to cosmetics because there are so many products on the market that are toxic. Here are some ingredients to steer clear of.

Top 10 Toxic Ingredients to Avoid in Cosmetics and your Personal Care products

Top 10 Toxic Ingredients to Avoid

1. Phthalates
2. Parabens
3. Sodium Laureth Sulfate (SLS)
4. Diethanolamine (DEA)
5. Triclosan
6. Synthetic Fragrance
7. Chemical UV filters - Octinoxate & Oxybenzone
8. Heavy Metals like Lead & Aluminum
9. PFOAs, PFCs and Teflon Chemicals
10. Petroleum and Mineral Oil

in Cosmetics & Personal Care Products

1. Phthalates - found in perfume, nail polish, hairsprays, shampoos and lotions-- these bad boys are actually a group of chemicals used to make products more flexible. In the past few

years, researchers have linked phthalates to asthma, attention-deficit hyperactivity disorder, breast cancer, obesity, type II diabetes, low IQ, neurodevelopmental issues, behavioral issues, autism spectrum disorders, altered reproductive development, and male fertility issues.

2.   Parabens - they're what make products last months or even years. Sounds great right? Not so much. Parabens are believed to disrupt hormone function by mimicking estrogen. As we know, too much estrogen can trigger an increase in breast cell division and growth of tumors, which is why parabens have been linked to breast cancer and reproductive issues, although the research isn't all there just yet. Do you mind paying to play the guinea pig? Didn't think so...

3.   Sodium Laureth Sulfate (SLS) - found in so many products that foam and suds up, SLS contains 1.4 Dioxane (a dangerous carcinogen) and is banned in Canada. You'll find it in face washes, shampoos, conditioners, hair dye, dental care products, creams, soaps, lotions, lip balms, foundations, makeup removers, and hand sanitizers. SLS is a skin irritant and should be rinsed off as soon as possible. So, don't get caught forgetting to wash off your makeup if you do choose to use it occasionally. It's also important to remember that there isn't very good science on how it may interact with other chemicals. Bear in mind, there are a growing number of products available advertised as SLS free. Wouldn't you

rather use something that will nourish your skin, as opposed to potentially irritate it?

4.   Diethanolamine – or DEA for short is actually banned in some countries. DEA, and its compounds, are skin irritants. In laboratory experiments, where there was exposure to high doses of said chemicals, they have been shown to cause liver cancers and precancerous changes in the skin and thyroid. Be on the lookout for DEA lurking in everything from sunscreens and moisturizers to shampoos and cleansers.

5.   Triclosan - wreaks havoc on your gut's microbiome and isn't just found in cosmetics but also in toothpaste and heaps of other consumer products. A study published in the journal Science Translational Medicine suggests that, due to the gut's alteration of its microbiotic population-- triclosan activates genes that govern inflammation and cancer growth, causing "adverse effects on colonic inflammation and colon cancer." According to the study:

One group of mice who were fed a diet laced with triclosan for three weeks ended up with low-grade inflammation of the colon and saw their garden of gut microbes become notably depleted. When researchers chemically induced inflammatory bowel disease in another group of mice, those exposed to real-world levels of triclosan suffered increased damage to the colon and more severe symptoms of colitis than did mice who weren't fed the chemical.

Finally, in mice made to develop colon cancer, those exposed to triclosan at normal human levels developed more and larger tumors, fueled by the activation of genes known to drive the cancer's growth. In addition, these mice were slightly more likely to die of colon cancer than their counterparts whose diets and environments were triclosan-free.

The mice also suffered a significant decrease in their *Bifidobacterium*, friendly bacteria which had been shown to lower inflammation. Although the FDA has stated Triclosan is "not generally recognized as safe and effective," manufacturers continue to use it. So, keep your eyes peeled!

6. Synthetic Fragrance - According to the Environmental Working Group, the average fragrant contains about 14 secret chemicals that aren't listed on the label, many of which are respiratory irritants and neurotoxic. They are also linked to hormone disruption and allergic reactions. Manufacturers often use these chemicals simply because they work well to disperse the fragrance into the air and cause it to linger (12). These chemicals also help to cheaply recreate the desired scent (13). By all accounts, the fragrance industry is primarily self-regulated. According to the Invisible Disabilities Association:

The fragrance industry has traditionally been a very secretive industry. For decades secrecy was required to protect fragrance formulas from being copied by others. Fragrance formulas are

257

considered "trade secrets" and do not have to be revealed to anyone, including regulatory agencies.

7. Chemical UV filters like Octinoxate and Oxybenzone – If it's been shown to cause coral bleaching, it's probably not your best friend. Not only has Hawaii banned the stuff in their SPF, common UV filters are also known endocrine disruptors, suspected to interact with sex hormones, fertility and thyroid. In CDC data, researchers discovered a link between its exposure and low testosterone in adolescent boys. So, please, spare the children! While, at the National Institute of Health, scientists found Oxybenzone to increase the risk of developing endometriosis. Fortunately, you can feel confident slathering on zinc oxide, if you are concerned about sun exposure.

8. Heavy Metals like Lead & Aluminum – How about a dose of lead with that sultry red lipstick? Yup, you read that right. In a study back in 2012, the FDA tested hundreds of different lipsticks from 20 popular name brands. They discovered lead in ALL of them. Manufacturers don't even have to disclose the presence of lead, but lead is so toxic to the nervous system that there is NO safe level of exposure. Why would it be banned in household paint but still be allowed to stain that gorgeous pout? I would much rather pucker up for some extra-virgin coconut oil, thank you very much.

As far as aluminum is concerned, I recommend steering clear of it, at all costs. Some may argue this point, but it has been found in

Alzheimer's brains and could also contribute to a whole host of brain dysfunctions, including Parkinson's and neurological disease. It might also lead to breast cancer. As an ingredient devised to wick moisture and create a matte finish, you'll frequently find it in makeup and antiperspirant. I was shocked to discover it in a pricy liquid foundation someone gifted to me—as soon as I stopped using it, my pores improved. So, check labels, check labels, check labels.

9. PFOAs, PFCs and Teflon Chemicals – It took a long, long time for the FDA to finally ban PFOAs (I highly recommend watching *The Devil We Know* for all the gut-wrenching facts), but they were replaced with PFCs, which are likely just as bad, or worse. PFOAs are already found in nearly 100% of the entire human species. And now, our planet has been introduced to more of these "fluoro" ingredients, which should all be avoided like the plague… Unless, of course, you're into developing liver problems, kidney disease, uterine polyps, cancerous tumors, immuno-deficiency, etc. The list goes on! Yeah, I think we'll pass… Be sure to check all your makeup, cookware, fabric protectors and creams.

10. Petroleum and Mineral Oil- These days, it's nearly impossible to find a medicine cabinet without "Petroleum Jelly." You'll see it proudly advertised in diaper ointments, lotions and balms as "healing" to the skin. However, it can actually prevent skin from healing by drying it out and blocking pores. Researchers in a 2011 study in *The Journal for Women's Health* found that

mineral oil contains toxic hydrocarbons. Accumulating in female body fat, they also found it in breastmilk, leading them to state that "mineral oil hydrocarbons are the greatest contaminant of the human body." As a sludgy byproduct of the oil industry, it's a far cry from being sustainable or eco-friendly. So how can companies claim it to be "healing"? Well, because it creates a non-breathable plastic wrap type film on the skin, of course! Ok captain, I'll let you decide if you think it's worth keeping in that medicine cabinet of yours.

Ladies! Why must we expose our internal ecosystems to this nonsense? Short answer? We don't have to! There are such better alternatives to the onslaught of slyly marketed "beauty" junk food. Let's ditch this toxic sludge and get acquainted with the incredible power of Mother Nature.

With the help of our handy dandy EWG app, we can easily look up products and thus curtail a multitude of horrifying chemical side effects. Check out the Environmental Working Group website for fascinating articles www.ewg.org Their app is a great resource for scoring products 1-10 (or A-F). I know it's hard to part ways with some of your favorites so here's a good rule of thumb to start:

1. If 7 or above REPLACE
2. If 4-7 RUN OUT
3. 1-3 ROCK ON!

It's also important to note, beyond lacking adequate data to understand the full effect of these chemicals, we lack adequate data to help illuminate how the myriad of chemicals interact with one another. For example, **one** such interaction that *was* researched-- between number four on our list (DEA) and nitrosamines-- found an unsavory chemical side effect. Scientists discovered that DEA compounds react with nitrites (which occur when preservative-laden cosmetics are exposed to air), forming *nitrosamines.* The International Agency for Research on Cancer classifies nitrosamines as a possible human carcinogen. That's just a glimpse into how TWO chemicals can react with one another. Imagine all the chemical interactions that have not been tested—not only between two separate chemicals, but between three, four, five, eighty-eight, and so on.

To add insult to injury, most beauty products come in "convenient" plastic packaging. Not only is the industry's addiction to plastic harmful to the environment, plastic packaging can also leach into the product itself. By now, your head might be spinning (even if you already unplugged that Glade). So, take a deep breath. There is a magical, wonderful world of natural products and DIYs awaiting your fingertips.

I also simplify the journey and give you a 'Done for You template' if you like that kind of approach in my online programs.

To learn more, check out the Resources page on my website.

Chapter 12: Your Physical Recovery, Sleep, Self-Love and Self-Care

First off, if you don't have one date scheduled with yourself on a regular basis, to self-care and self-love, you have a boundary issue and are likely codependent in some way. That takes a lot of work to dissect and is the kind of work I do that extends far beyond the pages of this book, but for now, let's dive info some common questions that will help you with some immediate attention.

Self-care for Explant Warriors

Scar Treatment

What to do about these explant scars? First, I want to say this: I actually have learned to love my scars and asked my partner at the time to massage them with love so I can feel them and thank them for the lessons they have taught me and what they represent. They are our "battle wounds" and the price we pay for being a student of life, learning how not to live, and learning what "self-love" truly is.

That said, there is a way to minimize them and ultimately heal them emotionally, as behind every scar, there is usually an unprocessed memory and trapped trauma that gets buried, later to arise as projected, and misdirected anger. It's *so* important to consider both the physical and emotional aspects of what scars represent to us.

Scar Healing Serum: For the physical scar, I put together a scar serum – a blend of frankincense, melaleuca (tea tree), helichrysum and yarrow palm diluted with vitamin E and jojoba oil. Almond oil is also nice for scars and smells sweet too. You can add a few drops of peppermint because it is soothing to the skin.

You can also include lavender or Neroli as individual oils, which are also known to reduce scarring. Remember not to overdo it, little bits, more often is better. The roller balls can be *very* handy and easy to throw in your purse or travel with since they are already pre-blended with the essential oil base and carrier oil. The kinds I recommend, and use are in my Resources section.

I have other products I can recommend too, but these have been super effective in my healing. I can barely even notice them now... But I'm also not hyper focused on them either … And am actually proud of them.

When Will My Hair Grow Back?

Everyone says "have your thyroid checked" which is *partially* helpful, but it is a) only a tiny piece of the picture and b) nearly 100% of the doctors don't run a *full* thyroid panel on you. It doesn't reference BII but what we say is that we don't "specialize" in any one disease or symptom. We work on teaching you to self-heal and strengthen your roots in your gut, brain and hormones so all

263

your symptoms, hair loss being one of them, cease to exist. Generally, hair loss is hormones, gut and toxicity-- as is everything.

Your Guide to the Best Beauty Sleep Ever

Are you ready to count unicorns instead of smelly sheep?

Basic Sleep Optimization Recommendations			
No screens 90 min before bed		Sleep in total silence	
No bright lights 90 min before bed		Sleep in total darkness	
Natural dim light for bedroom		Read an uplifting book before bed	
No caffeine after 10am		Work "In" before bed	
Binaural beats		Avoid intense exercise after dinner	
Avoid sugar/refined grains at night		Download f.lux on your computer	
Diaphragmatic breathing before bed		Temperature in bedroom 70 or below	
No phones in/near the bed		Warm/hot bath before bed (Epsom Salt)	

Basic sleep optimization recommendations:

Sleep is *king,* or shall I say *queen.* If you're not feeling your best, the first thing to question is "How am I sleeping?" You shouldn't wake up to pee in the middle of the night, contrary to common statements like "but I drink so much water," nor should you toss and turn. Before you pop that Xanax, consider all of the amazing alternatives to help you count sheep or unicorns or whatever spirit animal it is that sparks your imagination and melatonin to slip into dreamland.

Here's an extensive list of all your options:

No Screens – The blue/white light from TV, phone, computer, tablet, etc. … screens (as well as from bright light bulbs) will inhibit the production of melatonin (sleep hormone) and increase cortisol (stress hormone), negatively impacting your ability to fall asleep, and stay asleep. It is recommended by most sleep experts to avoid the screens for at least 90 minutes before going to bed. Once the sun goes down, we're supposed to wind down with it, even in winter when the sun goes down at 5 p.m. What do you think our ancestors did? They hibernated, of course.

Natural Lights – Certain colors of light actually increase melatonin production at night, and those are orange/red lights (like fire). The best option for nighttime light (in your bedroom or around the house) is Himalayan salt lamps. I absolutely love these and recommend having at least two in your bedroom. (Enough light to read by if they're on the nightstands/close to the bed) They are also said to purify the air, which is an added bonus.

Diffuse Essential Oils

Essential oils combat mold microorganisms decrease the toxicity of chemicals and increase atmospheric oxygen. They do all of this while leaving your home smelling great! A great trade in for Glade plug-ins and Febreeze, two of *the* most toxic products Americans buy for their homes to "smell better," which wreaks havoc on our sinuses, so invariably we're left "smelling worse" …

Through our own noses that is. I diffuse oils all day, and I recommend you do this while recovering from surgery so you're always breathing in light, love, and longevity.

Lavender has been shown to promote relaxation and better sleep, as well as lowered blood sugar while decreasing the production of stress hormone, cortisol in another study.

Other Sleep hacks

- Binaural Beats
- ASMR
- Deep Belly Breathing
- Meditation
- Yoga Nidra
- My current favorite for insomnia is Emotional Freedom Technique (EFT). Most people can learn this gentle tapping technique in several minutes.

Invest in an air purifier, especially if you or someone in your home snores. The quality of the air we breathe impacts the quality of our sleep more than we are programmed to think. Today's air is very toxic and even if you live in a rural area with a 'safe' score, the toxins we use in our own home off gas enough for the mucosa in our lungs and sinuses to rebel against us. I have one at home myself, it's listed in my Resources section.

Sleep in complete darkness or as close as possible. When light hits the eyes, it disrupts the circadian rhythm of the pineal gland and disturbs production of melatonin and serotonin. There also should be as little light in the bathroom as possible if you get up in the middle of the night. No TV right before bed. Even better, get the TV out of the bedroom or even out of the house, completely. It is too stimulating to the brain and it will take longer to fall asleep. It also disrupts pineal gland function, for the same reason as above.

Wear socks to bed. Due to the fact that they have the poorest circulation, the feet often feel cold before the rest of the body. A study has shown that this reduces night waking's. Bonus to apply essential oils such as Cedarwood, Frankincense or Lavender to your feet beforehand.

Read something spiritual, uplifting, self-loving or religious. This will help you to relax. Don't read anything stimulating, such as a mystery or suspense novel, as this may have the opposite effect. In addition, if you are really enjoying a suspenseful book, you might wind up unintentionally reading for hours, instead of going to sleep.

Avoid using loud alarm clocks. It is very stressful on the body to be woken suddenly. Instead, set a calming one.

Journaling. If you often lay in bed with your mind racing, it might be helpful to keep a journal and write down your thoughts before bed.

Get to bed as early as possible. Our systems, particularly the adrenals, do a majority of their recharging or recovering during the hours of 11 p.m. and 1 a.m. In addition, your gallbladder dumps toxins during this same period. If you are awake, the toxins back up into the liver which then secondarily back up into your entire system and cause further disruption of your health. Prior to the widespread use of electricity, people would go to bed shortly after sundown, as most animals do, and which nature intended for humans as well.

Be mindful of how much water you drink before going to bed. Additionally, use the bathroom before you lie down to sleep. This will reduce the likelihood of needing to get up and go to the bathroom or at least minimize the frequency.

Take a hot bath, shower or sauna before bed. When body temperature is raised in the late evening, it will fall at bedtime, facilitating sleep.

Aim to wind down around the same time every night. You should go to bed, and wake up, at the same times each day, even on the weekends. This will help your body to get into a sleep rhythm and make it easier to fall asleep and get up in the morning.

Sleep is queen, sister and your body will need all the help you can get, now and post explant!

Chapter 13 - booby traps ahead! The #1 thing you need to avoid 'falling off'.

So now that you've come to the final chapter, you're probably feeling excited... And a bit overwhelmed! For better or worse, transformation is not information. To simply store this whole book in your mind, without utilizing any part of it, would be a travesty. Now it's time to get motivated-- and that's what we're here for! By all means, change does NOT happen overnight. We cannot plant a seed then wake up the next morning to see a mature cherry blossom tree in full bloom. You need to water that seed, give it water, fresh air and plenty of sunshine!

This book has given you the seed, but now it's time for you to plant it. Each day you delay, is more time lost to fulfil your inner soul's prophecy to witness your tree's full potential. If the Covid-19 crises has taught us anything, it's that our health is FIRST and foremost our OWN. Our daily actions affect our overall health outcomes. We want to enjoy optimum well-being to avoid resorting to urgent care or an emergency room. There's never an ideal time to be sick but if we're healthy, our chances of having to go to a hospital during a dangerous time in history, is greatly diminished.

The viral scare has shown us the importance of looking out for our own preventative health, which is not what Western medicine does... Neither the FDA, nor the American Medical Association protected us with long-term studies on breast implants, Botox, various medical devices, or countless other chemicals readily available on the market.

269

Since no doctor in the world can do your shopping for you, serve you breakfast, lunch and dinner, your health is truly in your own hands. Take back the power and responsibility of honoring your vessel to its fullest potential. Trust your own instincts-- because you are not a lab rat. There will never be a lab rat with your name who has owned your biology or lived your life.

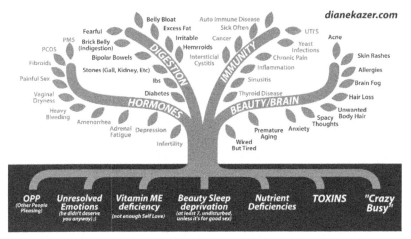

The road to illness begins with many roots. The path to wellness succeeds when you address them all!

BOOBY TRAPS ahead!

So, what are some of the obstacles you may have implementing the formula outlined in this book? The number one thing I see is women shaming and victimizing themselves. You may catch yourself overusing the following statement: "Oh, but my _____ !!!" (Insert dis-ease in the blank-- such as Lyme, Hashimoto's, fibromyalgia, allergies, etc.) This is a mistake! You are unintentionally owning a mindset that you are victim to the disease or a victim to your breast implants themselves. Try to remove statements like this from your mind. Moreover, do not allow such statements to exit your lips. Your ego subconsciously attaches itself to potentially damaging beliefs or myths, slowing down your healing process. These "booby traps" are the PRISON BARS that keep you from planting the seeds of your healing process.

Watch out for the following Booby Trap Myths, summarized throughout this book and below:

MYTHS

1. Breast implants are the reason for ALL my symptoms and explant is going to solve ALL my health problems. All my symptoms are going to miraculously go away after explant.

   o TRUTH = there are three main reasons why people develop chronic illness today: toxicity, infections, and trauma. Given this, breast implants are just 1 source of toxicity and infection... There are many other reasons to consider when the body is breaking down. We need to address all sources of stress on the body, not just one.

2. The body detoxes heavy metals, silicone and saline all by itself. I don't need to do anything other than remove my breast implants because it will take care of itself in time. Time heals all things.

   o TRUTH = It typically takes 1-2 years of being very intentional about healing the body with an approach that is unique to you. In general, we need to focus on properly detoxing the body, restoring immune function, healing the gut, and actively practicing mental/emotional detox. Those who miss any of these crucial stressors likely won't realize their full potential.

3. My breast implants aren't causing me any problems. My breasts look and feel fine.

o   TRUTH = Illness caused by implants are a conglomerate of 80+ symptoms such as brain fog, depression/anxiety, skin issues, hair loss, weight gain, pain, inflammation, chronic fatigue, autoimmune disease, frequent infections, GI symptoms, low body temp/blood pressure, infertility and more! You may have symptoms that you've labeled as "normal" or a part of getting older that could be partially connected to your breast implants. Like we always say in my practice, we can't blame every symptom on breast implants, but they certainly are a stressor on the body even if you think you're healthy. If you struggle with any symptoms, we always recommend removing the implants while also addressing any other hidden stressors. Why wait until you're really suffering? At any point, your breast implants could become a problem if the "perfect storm" situation presents itself.

4.   My body can't detox because I have the MTHFR genetic mutation.

o   TRUTH = Your genetics are impacted by your environment (lifestyle, toxic exposures, medications, stress, diet, mindset, thoughts and beliefs). These things can "dirty" your genes, meaning they can turn gene mutations "on" or "off" depending on how these factors are interacting with your body and affecting gene expression. This is called epigenetics. Clean up your environment and your body and your genes don't have to ruin your life. I've worked with plenty of women with the MTHFR gene mutation (including myself) with no issues.

5.   Chlorella, cilantro, and spirulina are good binders for detoxing heavy metals post explant surgery.

o   TRUTH = These are very weak binders and can end up doing more harm than good. I've seen these types of things make people much

272

sicker. Because they are weak binders, they often let go of toxins before they're ever even close to being eliminated from the body, and when that happens, toxins are driven even deeper into the tissues, including the brain. So, for very toxic individuals, I would caution to stay away from these weak binders. Using strong binders like we do in our program is imperative for restoring health. I would also caution against using most zeolites or clinoptilolite products on the market because when third party tested, almost all of them have been found to be contaminated with heavy metals (including TRX), and because of that, are very diluted. And in addition, using products like this without supporting all the detox pathways will eventually lead to a crash.

6.   I need to do a "candida cleanse" and/or "parasite cleanse" after explant to heal my gut.

o   TRUTH = Pathogens are there for a reason, usually due to poor immune function caused by toxins and trauma. Going on a bug-killing spree will not address the reason they are there (weak immune function, hormonal chaos, etc.). You must heal the root cause to heal the entire body holistically. I've seen a number of women who try to address gut infections alone and it's never successful if heavy metal toxicity is still an issue. They need to be addressed together, while also restoring immune function and addressing mental/emotional toxicity.

7.   Every symptom I have after explant is a result of detox reaction.

o   TRUTH = Breast implants and most surgical devices cause our bodies a tremendous amount of stress and destruction that require deeper healing than simply removing the source. Some symptoms can be detox related, yes. But more often than not, the symptoms that linger post-explant are a result of several factors: you just underwent a very aggressive and stressful surgery and it takes time for the body to recover from that; your detox pathways have completely shut down and your body is struggling to get rid of toxins effectively; there are other hidden stressors that still need to be addressed; you haven't dealt with underlying mental/emotional stressors (this will prevent you from healing).

8. I need tons of lab work to reveal my health issues.

o TRUTH: Proper lab work can cost a fortune! Oftentimes, if we put our focus on the three most common root causes of chronic illness, the body will get back into a state of normal function without needing all the lab work. If we run into road-blocks along the way, that's where some lab work can be helpful. I prefer to put my money where it counts most… An actionable plan. Additionally, most doctors (including naturopathic doctors) are not properly trained on how to explore the deepest root cause issues for why you're sick. You may have experienced a situation where you ask your doctor for lab work and the results are all "normal". That's because they aren't trained on how to read between the lines and interpret lab work from a functional perspective. The reference ranges for blood work were not created from a pool of healthy people, but rather a combination of both sick and healthy. Averages of this pool are considered "normal" but sadly, "average" is far from "normal." Bottom line: if you're going to do lab work, you want it analyzed with a fine-toothed comb.

9. I don't need any support to detox.

o TRUTH = In order to address EVERY facet of your healing journey, it's imperative to understand that you need to utilize your resources in an intelligent way. If your methods contradict each other, you could be back at square one. A single individual does not contain ALL the answers, and that's OK! It's OK to have help and structure that help into your daily life. Most of the time, we walk around with roadblocks chained around our necks and we don't even know that they're there-- or what they are! These roadblocks may be specific to you and you alone. A professional will help illuminate these roadblocks and customize an approach tailored to your individual healing journey.

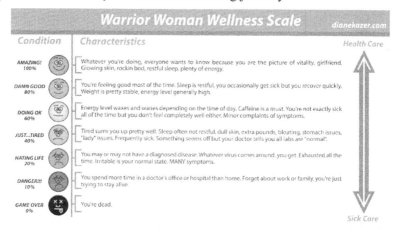

These are the "Talk Sick" Stories, beliefs, excuses that cause women to give up and go from maybe 30% of their full potential to 50-60%-- which could be two times better, and where most are still just feeling ok. Here is where women get deceived. Unfortunately, it's also where most of them quit, since although they feel better, they aren't thriving as their best selves. It's where they'll fly under the radar. This is also a "neutral" danger zone because lack of symptoms doesn't equate to health. Many will easily get sick or knocked off of their "feeling better" zone with one exposure to a bad bug, chemical, argument or life challenge-- such as a job change, move, death, break up, etc.

When I start working with a new patient, my CHI program focuses on these THREE PILLARS:

CLEANSE

- Detox - People often quit when they experience detox symptoms. This is because they fear them since they don't understand them. My goal is to help them understand what their symptoms mean and alleviate the root cause.

HEAL

- What are the core wounds holding me back from living my best life? How can I get "unstuck" and reclaim my health? Where can I support my hormones and gut at the root of their imbalances?

IGNITE

- Our beliefs, values, etc. that held us back must shift in order to help us perform at our optimum level. That way, we are motivated to continue up leveling our wellness lifestyle.

- For the average American, 70% of our day is spent in fight or flight mode. This perpetuates hyper focus on the body - OCD - body dysmorphia. Let's shift this hyper focus to hyper-self-love.

Phases of Spiritual Evolution on the Warrior Women Path

When you begin to awaken, your intuition communicates to the mind... "Something isn't right, what's going on with my life? Why am I not happy?" When you call in empowerment and evolution, you seek opportunities for growth. As you do, you move through these steps, this continuum, what I believe will FREE us from the prison cell in which we live. Each step diffuses yet another bar, until we are bar-less, disease-less and ultimately, limit-less.

1. **STEP 1** - We begin with awareness. We realize our starting point. Up until this point, we have just been "DEALING" with life, people pleasing, and acquiring prison bars from others.

2. **STEP 2** - To cope, we mindlessly start STEALING energy from others, food, our future self (we even steal resources from our body by catabolism - aka aging).

3. **STEP 3** - Then we move into the PEELING phase. We begin to peel back the layers of false self/ego and expose the root causes of fear/shame/guilt.

4. **STEP 4** - After that comes FEELING, and we begin to walk through the emotions of our past, ones that were *suppressed* yet never *addressed* and that consequently made us *depressed*.

5. **STEP 5** - We begin to move into a state of HEALING whereby we are able to repair parts of self that have suffered for years as a consequence of Step 2.

6. **STEP 6** - We get REAL. We become REAL. We live in truth and are often referred to as "the real deal." This is where the REAL MAGIC begins.

This explant journey is a form of Awakening, and it's a powerful one. Ultimately, it's important you have support through it all, because you've probably been there before when you go about it alone:

You FALL OFF

Feel GUILTY

Live in SHAME

PUNISH yourself (self-attack = auto-immune disease)

BURY the pain

GET SICK, feel like CRAP

Doctors' Visits, Expensive Labs, No Answers. You get FRUSTRATED

You Go Broke

You Give Up

You Get MORE sick...

Let me ask you:

Do you want to be free?

How bad do you want it?

How long can you afford your soul and life's purpose to ferment in the "dealing" phase? You are not here to people please or meet the expectations of others. You are here to please yourself, fulfil your purpose with your God-given gifts to change the mother f*cking world, warrior!

You are here to plant a beautiful new you, with healthy roots, a strong trunk, supportive branches and vibrant, glowing leaves. I cannot wait for you to start this journey and offer my helping hand, however I can.

Chapter 14 – Conclusion

Let's pull it all together.

You can do one of three things with this information.

#1 You can do nothing

#2 You can implement them on your own

#3 You can work with a practitioner and coach to help guide you along the way toward your wellness.

#4 You can do #3 with the intention of learning to become a health coach to yourself so you can then teach the formula to support women who are seeking the very advice you are right now.

You get to decide.

I find the greatest gift in all of this is being able to help others on their journey where like me at one point, and you right now, are lost, seeking guidance and a light on the windy path back to our happy selves, healthy body and whole heart.

I put loads of information to support you in the Resources section of my website, here are some quick links:

o   My home page: www.dianekazer.com

o   Talk to me: www.dianekazer.com/call

o   Resources Section: www.dianekazer.com/resources

Your fire of passion within can go one of two ways: Inflame your body or Ignite your purpose! My theory is:

Set fire to your dreams, not your body!

Your soul goal, when unexpressed festers within, causing inflammation.

Your purpose, when expressed outwardly, ignites your life!

Playing small is literally one of the greatest causes of illness of all...and I don't mean your breasts. You went big with those once, remember where that got you!

Thank you for your trust in me to read 'Killer Breasts' all the way through, your love for yourself, your belief in your purpose and your dedication to your wellness.

I am honored you chose me as your guide and I hope one day, we have the chance to hug, Silicone free, and heart to heart.

With CHI light and love towards your liberation!

Diane Kazer

P.S. I'll see you in the next book, which is already in motion.

It is my belief that breast implants are a part of the transhumanism agenda, which I am not a fan of. It is a cultural movement supporting the use of science and technology to improve human mental and physical characteristics. The movement regards aspects of the human condition, such as disability, suffering, disease, aging, and involuntary death as unnecessary and undesirable. Transhumanists look to biotechnologies and other emerging technologies for these purposes.

I'll tell you one thing, the day I removed my breast implants was the day I woke up and out of this spell, and my whole life changed. I sought truth and discovered my authentic power, my life purpose and an inner strength I never had before. I lost fear and gained love. Traded anxiety and worry in for peace and confidence.

If these are on your vision board, follow me through the plastic portal into the divine dimension where natural beauty and abundance thrive before you. It is happening now, and my vision is to take you there... so you may fall in love with yourself, your journey and your everything.

Stay in touch and stay tuned!

Supplement Recommendations

One of the top questions I am asked is 'What Supplements should I take?' and my answer is always 'it depends'. When I first started this journey and researched this question, I found a list of over 125 supplements, which blew my mind. I thought "My clients are overwhelmed when I recommend ten supplements, let alone 125". That was when one of the voices in my head said "We have to help these ladies. They need a simplified version of this as well as a customized option".

So here we are!

Perhaps the 2.0 version of this book will have more polished and professional images, but for now, behold my supplement triangle of hierarchy, from Staples to Specialty support.

I work with women who have BII as well as hormone imbalances, gut disfunction, trapped trauma and PTSD, toxic shame, toxic beauty symptoms, and more, so this will vary for every treatment protocol, however in BII, here is the simplified outline of what I generally recommend. These protocols should be done in phases, usually in months, so as not to take too many pills at once, nor overwhelm the body.

It is absolutely imperative before you embark on any supplement journey that you calm your Central Nervous system, balance your brain and strengthen your Vagus Nerve such that you reduce any fight or flight, that way your body does not reject these supplements, but rather receives them.

A few rules of thumb on supplements:

1. Be sure to titrate up to tolerance. I.e. if the bottle says take two twice per day, start with one pill, one time, then work up to four total.

2. Take only high-quality supplements that ensure testing so that you know you are getting what you are paying for.

3. Purchase supplements that maximize absorption rate. Such as liposomal Vitamin C vs Citric acid.

4. I wouldn't waste your time buying supplements at the store. First off, the clerk at the store, as well intended and informed as they may be, has not seen your medical history, nor labs, nor is a BII expert. Second, stores are only able to sell the low doses levels of supplements. This may not suit your nutritional needs.

5. Your best bet is to have your supplement protocol customized to you considering everything in this book to ensure you don't waste any more money than you need to on things you don't need. Explant surgery is expensive enough.

I see women who are on $500 per month protocols all the time, recommended by their functional medicine doctor. The supplements are usually high quality, but are not getting to the root of cellular toxicity, gut dysbiosis, hormonal chaos and lymphatic congestion in the proper order.

While I cannot tell you exactly what to do, here is a great foundation to consider:

STAPLES:

- Spore Based Probiotics (species that seed the gut, no refrigeration needed)

- Adrenal and Thyroid Stress formula (with ingredients such as B6 as P5P, ashwagandha, licorice root, rhodiola)

- Liver and Gall Bladder Detox support (Preferably containing high levels of NAC, Lipoic Acid, Vitamin C)

- Beauty and Immunity Multivitamin to provide key nutrients for energy, mental health and vitality (with Zinc, minerals, MSM, Vitamin A, C, D, B vitamins, as well as Amino Acids such as Glycine, Lysine and Proline)

- Collagen Peptides Powder to add to smoothies or coffee to strengthen and repair internal tissues, skin, hair

CLEANSING:

In addition to the liver and gall bladder formula, you'll need deeper detox for:

- Systemic Enzymes for Lymphatic Decongestant and inflammation reduction

- Cellular Detoxification with Clinoptilolite Zeolites, phosphatidylcholine, fulvates and if you're working with a BII specific practitioner, EDTA

- Strong Binders with Magnesium Oxide, various fibers, Activated Carbon, Fulvic acid and Zeolites.

HEAL GUT & HORMONES

In addition to the Adrenal stress support and spore probiotics, I also recommend:

- Digestive support for the 5 R Protocol such as:
- o Remove - Antimicrobials, antifungals
- o Replace - Bitters, HCL, Digestive Enzymes
- o Repair - a Leaky Gut Repair formula, a Mucosal support blend.

- o Reinoculate – Spore Based Probiotics and saccharomyces boulardii (if fungal overgrowth present)
- o Rebalance – feed the probiotics with prebiotic formula

While you can take all of the supplements in order for the 5R protocol I've listed here, it makes far greater sense to have this customized concurrent with your labs, BII journey, symptoms, medical history, lifestyle and toxicity levels.

- Hormone Healing Protocol customized to your labs
- o Thyroid Glandulars
- o Adrenal Glandulars
- o Magnesium
- o DIM, CDG for Estrogen Dominance
- o Minerals for deficiencies and balance

RELIEF CARE

If you're experiencing symptoms of discomfort, until you can resolve the root cause, you might consider supplementing with:

- Sleep tonics (Cortisol managers)

- Pain modulators

- Neurotransmitter balancers and CNS regulators (5HTP, GABA, Sam-E, amino acid therapy, etc.)

- CBD

- Essential oils

I posted some options for you on the Resources page of my website.

Remember, proper heavy metal detox protocols, when done right, take one to two years.

Proper gut healing protocols, considering all phases take at least six months.

Hormone balancing protocols take three to six months.

There are also formulas to detox pesticides such as glyphosate from your body, but that is beyond the context of this book and is something I consider when working with one on one clients on a case by case basis.

The least overwhelming and most specific thing you can do is work with an expert practitioner who is familiar with BII and has extensive experience supporting women from start to finish, to support you with this and monitor your progress.

Remember: Healing begins in the mind and Detox is blocked with mental stress. And 60% of any pills efficacy is predicated on your thoughts about what it will do for you (placebo).

"Toxins trapped in the physical body are reflections of thoughts, fears, beliefs, stories and emotions that are held in the mental and emotional bodies. When you free the fear, surrender the stories and clear the mind from thoughts that traumatize you, your body automatically frees the toxins that create symptoms, sickness and suffering."

The important thing is to tell yourself a life story in which you, the hero, are the problem solver rather than the helpless victim. This is well within your power, whatever fate might have dealt you, and will be the master supplement to your supplement journey from BII to FLY (First Love Yourself).

A Success Story, Life After Explant

Where is Emily now?

"Dear Diane and CHI team,

At the onset of my long list of bizarre symptoms, functional medicine doctors diagnosed me with toxic mold sickness. I experienced acute exposure in a moldy house where we lived during the previous year while I was pregnant. I took the steps that the doctors insisted were necessary to rid myself of the mold but remained sick. That's when I began searching and found your team.

Post CHI gratitude – Thank you for helping me understand that my breast implants were distracting my immune system – preventing it from dealing with the mold. I had no idea that commonplace items in my everyday life were laden with toxins and drastically impacting my health. From pharmaceutical drugs, hormonal birth control, allergy meds, beauty products, cleaning supplies, Botox, glyphosate – and of course the mold. I was unknowingly poisoning myself and my family. Finally, the house of cards fell, and my health suffered greatly, as did my son's. Thanks for helping us both heal and for showing us a better way.

I'm now free from: Insomnia, Chronic fatigue, Muscle weakness, Full body pain, Unexplained weight loss, Heart palpitations, Depression, Anxiety, Explosive rage, Blurred vision,

Diarrhea, Constipation, Mast cell activation disorder, Food sensitivities Rosacea

Tinnitus (ear ringing) and mold toxicity.

I've gained 30 much needed pounds. My hair has stopped breaking off and falling out and my brain fog is getting better by the day. Best of all, my son's health issues have completely resolved, and he is thriving. Oh and no more night sweats! I used to SOAK my bed sheets and had to sleep on beach towels!"

WOW! Pretty powerful isn't it? Especially for Emily and most of us who have been there or are still there...you're not going crazy, you're not alone and you're not broken...our system is.

Imagine what would be possible for you, if you finally felt seen and understood, that your body is speaking to you, in the language of symptoms and it's dying to be heard and healed.

Symptoms are self-love from the Soul, all you need is a team or coach to help you decode what they mean so you can give your body exactly what it needs to come alive and

THRIVE...just like Emily did.

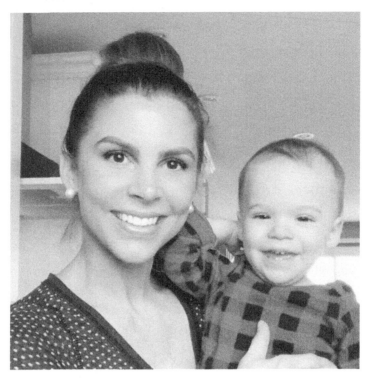

Emily and little Lyle, after their detox and gut restoration. All smiles!

Case Study

MY Reversing AUTO-IMMUNE Disease JOURNEY and how Functional Medicine labs SAVED me

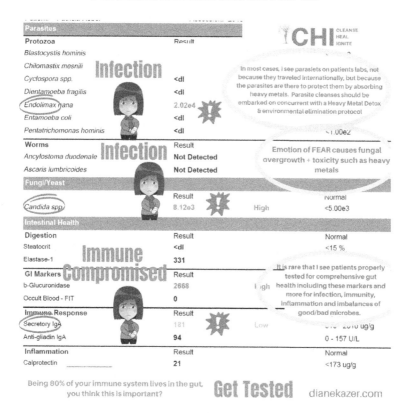

Being 80% of your immune system lives in the gut, you think this is important? **Get Tested** dianekazer.com

THYROID HEALTH VIA COMPREHENSIVE TESTING:

I self-diagnosed Hashimoto's after running my own thyroid labs 6 years ago to discover what multiple doctors did not, because while they 'tested my thyroid', they didn't test it completely. It's common practice, as I have seen in helping hundreds of women through hormonal, gut, mood and BII symptoms over the last decade, that they only test TSH, T3, and

T4, maybe Free T3 and T4, but they miss the antibodies, because Western medicine doctors are not trained that over 95% of Hypothyroid disease is caused by antibodies, they are taught it's the other way around (per the work of Dr Isabella Wentz, Thyroid Expert). AND according to my friend Dr Tom O'Bryan, it takes, on average, 10-15 years before one is properly diagnosed with auto-immune disease based on the current Western medicine model and testing, which means they can ONLY catch it once it happens rather than explore predictive lab markers before it surfaces as a full-blown disease. Logically, wouldn't it make sense to test for an impending disease, symptomatically and with proper labs so you can prevent it before it happens? This is why I check for these things in my clients, the moment they feel something is 'off', which is exactly what I found in my own labs.

GUT HEALTH VIA STOOL TESTING:

These were my results one year prior to removing my breast implants. Discovering what my bad ass body looked like inside, fighting to protect and keep me safe for nearly 10 years, dropped me to my knees in tears, holding it, apologizing to it for cutting it open, tearing it apart in the name of 'beauty'. Seeing the state my immune system was in and meeting the warrior inside of me that went to battle to beat the bugs that were there because the boob bags were, played a major role in my decision to remove them. Reason being, that for 6 years I had been on a gut healing protocol, including removing the bad bugs such as candida, bacteria and parasite overgrowth. After testing myself with these advanced functional medicine labs we use in my practice, I tracked the pattern back every year for 6 years and to my shock, the pathogens had not budged one bit. I had chronic critters inside of me that no amount of gut protocol would remediate. I have not done any scientific testing to explore if this was a parasite, candida or silicone, however my intuition told me it was silicone, because I have seen parasites come out of my stool and this is not what it looked like.

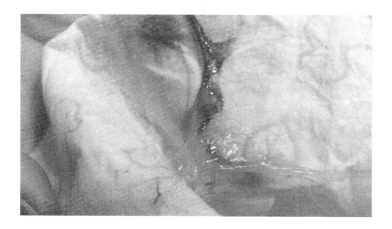

Once I learned that toxins taking up permanent residence in our body perpetuate them, it was an easy F*ck yes to explant. After spending hundreds of thousands of dollars on my body in attempt to heal, discovering that the root cause of it was living inside of me, it was like a light bulb went off and it illuminated my path toward silicone sovereignty. Since I've removed them, my symptoms have improved significantly, chronic disease no longer chronic, confirmed by my ever-improving labs I've tracked since D-Day aka explant day.

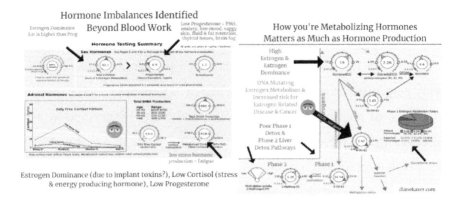

Breast Implants = Inflammation, Infection + Immune System Disfunction

Gut disfunction = Poor Immune health = Hormone Imbalance

Patient: Diane Kazer — Accession: 20180626-0224

Opportunistic Bacteria

Additional Dysbiotic/Overgrowth Bacteria	Result		Normal
Bacillus spp.	4.71e4		<1.50e5
Enterococcus faecalis	5.06e2		<1.00e4
Enterococcus faecium	<dl		<1.00e4
Morganella spp.	1.98e3	High	<1.00e3

Fungi/Yeast

	Result		Normal
Candida spp.	6.26e3	High	<5.00e3
Candida albicans	<dl		<5.00e2
Immune Response	Result		Normal
Secretory IgA	44	Low	510 - 2010 ug/g
Anti-gliadin IgA	173	High	0 - 157 U/L

Gold Marker SIgA low due to chronic stress trying to attack implants

GI Stool Testing via GI Map

HORMONAL HEALTH VIA URINE TESTING (before and after)

Estrogen Dominance (due to implant toxins?), Low Cortisol (stress & energy producing hormone), Low Progesterone

Above are my BEFORE results, 2 years prior to explant. My results 1 year before explant didn't look much different. As you can see, I had really low progesterone (which is Mother Nature's antidepressant), and higher estrogen relative to progesterone (Estrogen Dominance), as well as dangerously low Cortisol production. No wonder I was so tired, as Cortisol is our stress Hormone that helps us cope with stress, helps us discern aversion to a$$ holes (LOL), as well as are the fire-fighters in our

294

body that put fires of inflammation out, which is super characteristic to women suffering from BII.

On the second page here, the biggest concern I had seen consistent to all of my previous urinary hormone test results, was a dangerously high level of 4-OH-E1 (the # above you can see is 2.57). This is the dangerous estrogen metabolism pathway that increases damage to DNA and that level of mutation, increases odds of estrogen related disease and growth such as fibroids, cysts, tumors and cancer. Additionally, the first Phase of Liver Detoxification, is key to convert toxins, pharmaceuticals, hormones and things like xeno-estrogens, and it must be functioning optimally before Phase 2 Liver detox can take place. Both my phase 1 and 2 were in bad shape, as you can see my Methylation activity was Low, per my fan gage, akin to having an 'empty' tank of fuel in your vehicle.

LET'S TALK GENETICS FOR A SEC:

Of course, genetics DO play a role here as I am double Homozygous for the MTHFR 677 gene mutation, which can be overridden and biohacked with a healthy lifestyle, a peaceful mind and a body that is synced with nature. However, no matter how dialed in you are with all of those things, if you have breast implants, it can dirty that gene, causing it to act out and interrupt your Phase 2 detox pathways, backing your body up with toxins and hence sickness and symptoms. Add to that Botox, birth control, benzodiazepines, and a Bully in your head, and you've got a recipe for Disease disaster. There are also

FAKE BREASTS = FAKE ESTROGENS:

As you read in previous chapters, Xeno-estrogens are fake toxins that look like estrogen to the body so can occupy the receptor site, but aren't truly self-made, so it drives up levels of estrogen in the body (as seen on my lab tests). These aggressive toxins can out-compete our own made estrogen and can be up to 1,000 times more powerful, hence are a major threat to us all today, because they 'grow things' such as tumors, cysts, fibroids, endometrium, cancers, lymph nodes, fat cells (including the brain) contributing to the hormone imbalance, cancer, obesity and chronic illness epidemic today. The greater our exposure, the greater the impact. They are extremely powerful and are stored in our fat cells, which the brain is primarily comprised of. (Hello brain fog, confusion and mental disease)

Silicone is a Xenoestrogen. Don't forget that saline breast implants are cased in Silicone, so all implants contain Silicone. It's an endocrine (hormone) disruptor and displaces zinc in the body which is a precursor to progesterone, so it drives that down, which can cause estrogen dominance and estrogen dominance related conditions and symptoms. This is evident on my 'before and after' lab results which, as you can see my progesterone rose 1.27%, and I can absolutely feel it too! I have seen this with the women I have supported to and through explant in their mind, body, spirit recovery and rebuild. Aside from breast implants, sources of Xenoestrogens include plastics, pesticides, processed meats, packaged foods, parabens in beauty care products, phthalates in the ingredient 'fragrance', and water, The majority of filters do not adequately filter out prescription drugs such as birth control and run off from hormones used in agriculture, which is why I recommend having a whole house water filtration and drinking water system at home (see my resources page for more).

The overload and malabsorption of foreign estrogens can lead to a buildup of more "aggressive" proliferative forms of estrogen in the body. And when this happens, a whole host of health complications can ensue, including Breast Cancer. A study conducted at the University of Toronto found that women who ate muffins with 5 teaspoons of flax seeds per day were able to lower their tumor markers from 30-71%, as my dear friend, Veronique Desaulniers, the Breast Cancer Conqueror advises.

Additionally, she references "Because estrogen is involved in dozens of hormonal pathways in the body, the concern with Xeno-estrogen is also whether or not estrogen methylation in general is taking place in a healthy way. If your body is not able to metabolize or breakdown the chemical estrogens, then build-up and or estrogen dominance can occur. Another concern is how Xeno-estrogen interferes with not only the reproductive system (for both men and women - and children), but how it affects other cellular functions too. For example, Xeno-estrogen build-up can change brain chemistry and lead to neurological conditions. It can also cause imbalance in cortisol levels and thyroid hormone deficiency."

HERE ARE MY 'BEFORE' RESULTS AGAIN:

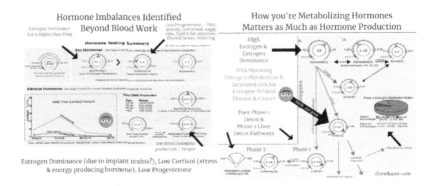

THE IMPROVEMENTS:

- SEX HORMONES INCREASED DRAMATICALLY
- PROGESTERONE SUPER HEALTHY LEVEL AND 227% HIGHER
- STRESS HORMONE CORTISOL PRODUCTION GREATLY IMPROVED BY 45%
- MASTER HORMONE DHEA PRODUCTION INCREASED 53%
- PHASE 1 LIVER DETOX GREATLY IMPROVED
- PHASE 2 LIVER DETOX WENT FROM LOW TO MID RANGE (AWESOME)
- STILL ESTROGEN DOMINANT (but that will improve over time as I clear the debris of Breast Implants, Botox and Toxic Beauty residue. Generally, it takes 1 month for every year you've had implants to cleanse and heal, which can be expedited if you work with a practitioner and run labs like these to explore healing opportunities and create a customized, accelerated protocol)

SO YOU CAN COMPARE THEM TO AND SEE THE DIFFERENCE IN MY 'AFTER' RESULTS:

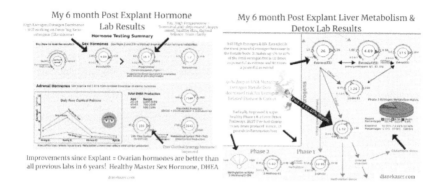

These results are truly remarkable, and it is thanks to the work of the many mentors who I have learned from over the years, that have helped me crate the Overcoming BII protocol in this book. It is my goal that every woman invest in her health in this way so she can experience the same!

Citations and Studies

https://dianekazer.com/33-reasons-not-to-get-breast-implants-your-doctor-didnt-warn-you-about/

https://www.plasticsurgery.org/news/press-releases/new-statistics-reveal-the-shape-of-plastic-surgery

https://www.fda .gov/medical-devices/breast-implants/risks-and-complications-breast-implants

http://web.archive.org/web/20040805034819/http:/implants.clic.net/tony/Blais/019.html

https://www.breastimplantillness.com/wp-content/uploads/2017/08/Mechanisms_of_Breast_Implant_Toxicity_By_Dr._Brawer251503803405105-1098318890.pdf

https://www.breastimplantillness.com/truth-cohesive-gel-implant/

http://web.archive.org/web/20031228073607/http:/implants.clic.net/tony/Blais/018.html

http://web.archive.org/web/20040804222605/http:/implants.clic.net/tony/Blais/008.html

https://clinmedjournals.org/articles/cmrcr/clinical-medical-reviews-and-case-reports-cmrcr-3-087.pdf

https://www.ncbi.nlm.nih.gov/pubmed/7570622

https://www.ncbi.nlm.nih.gov/pubmed/7855864

https://www.ncbi.nlm.nih.gov/pubmed/8565558

https://www.ncbi.nlm.nih.gov/m/pubmed/26264162/?i=1&from=silicone%20breast%20toxicity

https://www.bmj.com/rapid-response/2011/10/28/concerns-estrogenicy-silicone-breast-implants

https://www.ncbi.nlm.nih.gov/pmc/articles/PMC4036413/

https://juniperpublishers.com/crdoj/pdf/CRDOJ.MS.ID.555710.pdf

https://environmentalhealth.ucdavis.edu/endocrine-disruptors

https://www.accessdata.fda.gov/cdrh_docs/pdf3/P030053B.pdf

http://mybreastimplants.org/PDF/Original_07242007.pdf

https://www.ncbi.nlm.nih.gov/pubmed/9207676

https://www.ncbi.nlm.nih.gov/pubmed/16996440

https://www.ncbi.nlm.nih.gov/pubmed/7480245

https://www.ncbi.nlm.nih.gov/pubmed/7855864

https://www.ncbi.nlm.nih.gov/pubmed/7570622

https://www.youtube.com/watch?v=3JlAmYn_hws

https://www.ncbi.nlm.nih.gov/pubmed/12655204

https://www.ncbi.nlm.nih.gov/pubmed/21717259

https://www.plasticsurgery.org/for-medical-professionals/health-policy/bia-alcl-physician-resources?fbclid=IwAR1

UNxDw7A5UDOAp_DVj3gkoUZMaYaZ1fLi15OYe5bQnO4NjC-HZm3VUCDI

http://www.center4research.org/breast-implants-research-regulatory-summary/

https://www.ncbi.nlm.nih.gov/pmc/articles/PMC4366693/

http://www.center4research.org/breast-implants-research-regulatory-summary/

https://www.ncbi.nlm.nih.gov/m/pubmed/26264162/?i=1&from=silicone%20breast%20toxicity

Lynch, B. (2018) Dirty Genes. New York, NY: HarperOne

https://www.mayoclinic.org/tests-procedures/mammogram/expert-answers/breast-implants/faq-20057926

http://www.center4research.org/breast-implants-research-regulatory-summary/

https://www.sciencedaily.com/releases/2018/09/180917191649.htm

http://www.center4research.org/breast-surgery-likely-cause-breastfeeding-problems/

http://www.center4research.org/breast-implants/

http://www.center4research.org/breast-implants/

https://www.ncbi.nlm.nih.gov/pmc/articles/PMC4036413/

https://www.ourbodiesourselves.org/book-excerpts/health-article/facts-about-breast-implants/

https://journals.sagepub.com/doi/pdf/10.1177/1721727X1201000209

https://www.ncbi.nlm.nih.gov/pubmed/26218390

https://www.medicalnewstoday.com/articles/321610.php

http://www.center4research.org/breast-implants/

http://www.center4research.org/breast-implants/

http://www.center4research.org/breast-implants-research-regulatory-summary/

http://www.center4research.org/breast-implants/

https://20somethingfinance.com/percentage-of-americans-living-paycheck-to-paycheck/

Kolb, S.E. (2010) The Naked Truth About Breast Implants. Savage, MN: Lone Oak Publishing

https://www.breastimplantillness.com/wp-content/uploads/2018/01/Vague-Syndromes-.pdf

https://www.breastimplantillness.com/wp-content/uploads/2017/08/Mechanisms_of_Breast_Implant_Toxicity_By_Dr._Brawer251503803405105-1098318890.pdf

https://www.breastimplantillness.com/wp-content/uploads/2017/01/chronology-of-systemic-disease-development-in-300-symptomatic-recipients-dr.-brawer.pdf

https://www.womenshealthmag.com/beauty/a19910278/doves-choose-beautiful-campaign/

Special thanks:

To my science, spiritual and sovereignty mentors who have taught me much of what I included in this book (special thanks to Dr Tom O'Bryan, John McMullen, Dr Rick Malter, Reed Davis, Molly Meier, Maya Eller, Anna Rodgers, Dr Dan Pompa, Brene Brown, Marc VonMusser and my Auntie Andrea)

To my friends who held space for me in my moments of crumbling and cheered me on as I put myself back together again, especially Robbe Richman, who is 100% to blame for my Achilles tendon rupture.

To my magician friend, Jason Ring for waking me up and out of the matrix.

To my clients, like Emily, Amber, Lisa C, Genaye, Lauren, Lunden who trusted me to teach them the tools of transformation and to shine a light on their path back to their heart and purpose, who have shined that light back at me, through this journey, because f*ck, writing a book isn't easy!

To my surgeon, Dr Bradley Strawn, Sheena and all of the medical team for my explant procedure, rebuilding my breasts and caring for women the way you do!

To my partner, Functional Medicine MD, Dr Juan Manuel Garcia, expert in PRP, IV treatment, Stem cell therapy and post explant advanced healing

To my rescue dog, Kayla for rescuing me back and being a rock for me 24/7 through this whole experience, my greatest source of Oxytocin.

To the Divine, for always protecting me, and for gifting me the lessons I came here to learn.

To Mama Gaia, for reminding us what natural beauty is.

To my Creator, for giving me a great set of original tatas, that I couldn't see as beautiful the first time! I'm sorry for rejecting your idea of perfection, WTF do I know.

To myself, for having the COURAGE to share my most vulnerable moments, fear the unknown and do it anyway!

To my family for loving me through it all.

About the Author

Beyond the Boobs: From Silicone Suffering to Sovereignty & Self Love

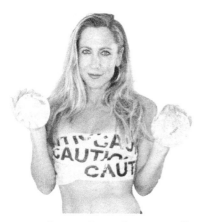

Diane Kazer is a Breast Implant Illness Recovery Expert, and author of Killer Breasts. She is the producer of the Non-Toxic Beauty Revolution and creator of CHI Hormone Warrior Transformation which offers women three pinnacles to wellness: "CLEANSE your body, HEAL your hormones, IGNITE your life". She has supported women in over 15 countries and earned the award as Orange County's top nutritionist and integrative health professionals. Though she has long been a visionary in the world of women's health, for 10 years Diane was sick – really sick – and hundreds of thousands of women everywhere are going through the same illness right now.

A pro soccer player in her early 20s, and bikini competitor, Diane's intense training kept her slim and toned – but flat-chested. Following breast implant surgery, she began to feel her body slowly change and spent years fighting mystery ailments. When she realized that the foreign material inside of her was toxic, and was slowly killing her, she took the necessary steps to remove them and regain optimal health. But she understood that explant surgery was only part of her journey, she needed to build an entire ecosystem of health around her that not only addressed the physical implications of both pre- and post-surgery, but also the mental and emotional implications – not the least of which is the deeply ingrained sense self-loathing that lead so many women to harmful cosmetic surgeries.

Knowing that there were hundreds of thousands just like her, women feeling isolated and alone as they fought Breast Implant Illness (BII), Diane made her mission to help women explore BII as a root cause for women's symptoms and suffering. She empowers women to heal themselves by addressing:

• Toxicity • Infection • Trauma • Shame

She helps women to reconnect to their divine purpose by activating and aligning their 4 Superpowers: Mind of the Sage, Temple of the Goddess, Spirit of the Unicorn, Heart of the Warrior. It is here where spirituality and self-love meet soul food and sisterhood. Her program, CHI, has empowered thousands of women to break free of the self-doubt that sabotaged them and the Toxic Beauty modifications that made them sick.

Disclaimer

I am Diane Kazer, and I am not an MD, nor do I diagnose or treat specific conditions. I always recommend you disclose your health concerns to your physician. Information in this book is shared as support for considerations and not medical advice. Diane and her business consultants do not endorse, recommend or suggest using any particular procedure, physician, or program mentioned in this book. All solutions discussed are for the convenience of the individual(s) receiving it to make their own informed personal decisions, based on the options provided.

Final Words

My wish for you is that you take this book and run with it until you FLY on your own. FLY meaning First Love Yourself. I wrote it as a self help'ish, but more so as a 'return to self love' book. It's said that the majority of people either don't finish or don't even start reading the books they buy, and I get it…it takes a lot of focus to sit down, read and actually focus today, especially with brain fog, which is so common in women with BII. If you read even parts of this book and found yourself saying…I love this, I get this and I want to learn how to do this…but I want to do it with the help of a coach who has 'been there, done that', I encourage you to reach out. There's nothing weak about asking for guidance, especially through this BII and Toxic Beauty journey. I was there once it was a huge challenge to do solo, without an expert by your side every step of the way, who has the 3 keys to help you help yourself transform – education, experience and empathy.

I WANT YOU TO KNOW YOUR HEART BECAUSE NOW, YOU KNOW MINE

Through the art of vulnerability, authenticity and my C.O.U.R.A.G.E. approach, I found my heart. I have shared it with you in this book, which is one of the scariest things I have ever done, but it's worth it because through my own hearts unveiling, now you may better and deeper know yours, which pays back divine dividends for life, and is what fuels me every day to know I am of service to you with this mission, helping you discover:

- How can I listen to my symptoms compassionately by learning the language of what they're trying to say, instead of shaming and numbing them?

- What's REALLY going on with my hormones and how do I fix them?

- How do I heal my gut so I can tune into my 'gut feelings' instead of gut discomfort?

- What sabotaging stories and limiting beliefs am I carrying around that keep me stuck and how do I free them?

- What is self-love? And how can I love others without losing myself?

When you heal each of these, you heal the whole of you.

Will you promise me something? After you've read this book, do 3 things:

- Leave a review (on Amazon or wherever you bought it).

- Share this book with women you know who need it.

- Drop me a line, and tell me how you're doing. My greatest wish is for you to be able to hug others closer to you now that those implants aren't blocking your heart. I would be honored to heart hug with you one day, after you've explanted, to celebrate your FREEDOM to FLY!

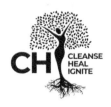

Visit www.DianeKazer.com to reclaim your inner CHI and natural beauty.

My mission is to educate and empower irrationally passionate women leaders with safer beauty, body and breast solutions from products and procedures to diet and detox, so they can age gracefully and holistically, with the energy and vitality they need to step into their power, speak their voice and spark their purpose!

I honor the place in you that is Courage, Compassion and Consciousness. I honor the place in you that is of love, light, truth and peace. When you are in that place in you, and I am in that place in me, we are one! NAMASTE!

Made in the USA
Monee, IL
05 March 2023

29197293R00184